THE RECOVERY TOOL BELT

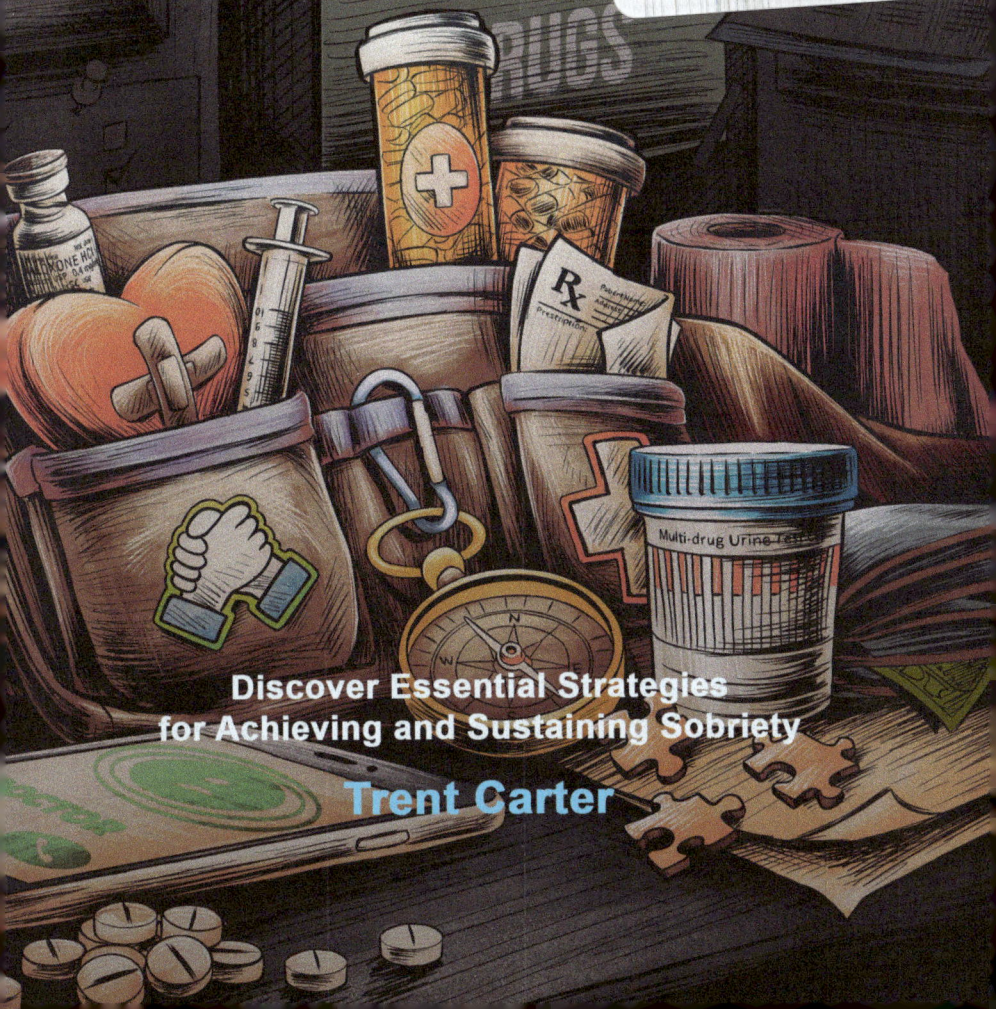

Discover Essential Strategies
for Achieving and Sustaining Sobriety

Trent Carter

ISBN: 978-1-956464-64-1

First Edition 2025

Published by BrightRay Publishing
https://brightray.com/

To my family, whose support and love have carried me through every challenge and triumph. Your love and belief in me drive me to be better each day.

To my patients, who have trusted me to walk this path with them. You teach me as much as I strive to teach you.

And to everyone who believes in building something brighter for those struggling with addiction. This book is for the fighters, the dreamers, and those daring to create a future where healing is possible for all.

TABLE OF CONTENTS

FOREWORD

This book is going to save lives and families. Having practiced medicine for nearly three decades, I have had the honor of caring for people in diverse settings, including primary care offices, emergency departments, crisis programs, and in a specialty addiction medicine and co-occurring mental health practice. As a physician and addiction medicine specialist, I am always seeking tools and pathways to help my patients and their loved ones navigate the journey to long-term recovery. *The Recovery Tool Belt* is what is needed.

Once I started reading *The Recovery Tool Belt*, I could not stop. My reaction was, "Finally, someone gets it." Yes, Trent gets it and has skillfully laid out a guide for people to start and, more importantly, continue their recovery journey. It has all the essential components to truly serve with the requisite balance between heart, science, clarity, and practicality.

I initially went into emergency medicine to make a big impact, to save lives. In addiction medicine, I believe we not only save lives but also help save families, businesses, and even communities. Addiction and recovery healthcare truly has a multi-generational effect. *The Recovery Tool Belt* will serve both the people seeking recovery and their loved ones.

Too often, patients or families seek care for substance use and addiction-related conditions but feel like they have nowhere to go. They may feel hopeless and overwhelmed by the consequences of the addiction, and are often plagued with shame and stigma. If substance use continues or if reuse/relapse occurs, it is too often treated with surprise and more shame as opposed to understanding, support, and positive re-engagement. Again, leading to more shame and hopelessness. People may experience learned helplessness and often feel broken or that something is irreparably damaged with their ability to make breakthroughs. However, the tools and methodologies for helping people with long-term, successful recovery are what is lacking. That is where *The Recovery Tool Belt* comes into play.

This book will guide people and empower hope. Not a blind, wishful hope but one based on heart and science. It encapsulates the three essential elements of hope: goals, a sense of agency, and pathways for progress. Recovery is not about perfection. It is about persistence and perseverance. Never giving up, and always continuing to engage. We stay engaged when we see possibilities. Overcoming many of our challenges often boils down to methodology, taking needed steps to help strengthen our abilities. But what is needed is a better understanding of the condition and how to take these steps. *The Recovery Tool Belt* breaks down this understanding and lays out the right steps.

I know, trust, and consult with Trent. He and this book are rare finds, and he is the kind of wellness and healthcare provider that people need. It is worth repeating that this book will save lives and families as well as help recovery specialists and other healthcare providers grow professionally.

I am a better addiction medicine physician after reading *The Recovery Tool Belt,* and I look forward to sharing it with my patients and colleagues.

– Dr. Drew C. Fuller, *BrightWell Health Medical Director, MD, MPH, FASAM, FACEP*

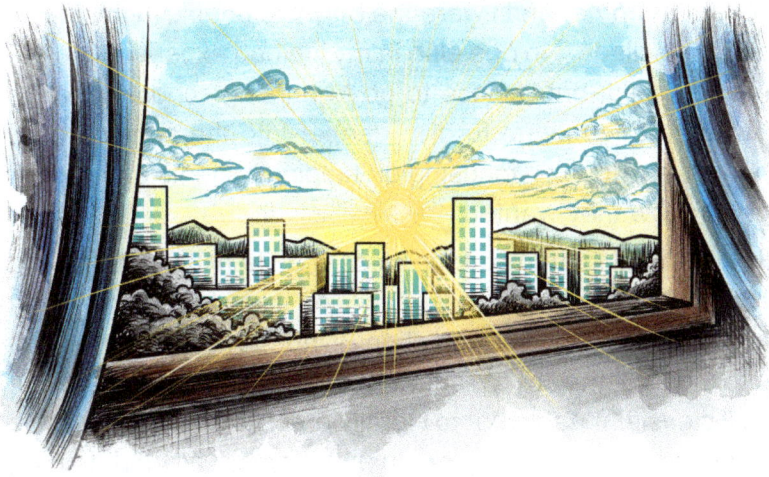

INTRODUCTION

Ever since I was young, I've been interested in the body and science. Growing up, I looked up to bodybuilders like Arnold Schwarzenegger, Ronnie Coleman, and Greg Plitt, fascinated by their ability to change their bodies and sculpt them how they wanted. As a young boy, whenever I found a subject I really liked, I would try to absorb everything, going as in-depth as I could. This was especially true with the sciences. I gravitated toward it because when faced with a problem, I could go through systematic steps to find out how something works and generate a solution. Often in life, there's plenty that we can't account for, and sometimes, we're left to settle with the best answer we can find. But in medicine, we have the ability to go through all the available processes and even create new processes so that we can fix people's lives and make things better, all by altering the body.

My older brother and I were the only two people in my family to go to college. No one else in my life had experience in the medical field, but I chose to go to nursing school because I wanted to continue to dive deeper into the subject that I had always loved—focusing on helping patients sculpt their health how they wanted.

I worked in many intensive care units (ICU) and trauma centers, and it was in these facilities that I had some of my first experiences with addiction. When an alcoholic comes into the ICU, they're typically not there to go into withdrawal, so it's easier for a doctor to literally prescribe them beer while treating them than to try and wean them off alcohol, forcing them into a detox they don't want. So for these patients, every six to eight hours, I'd go into a fridge and sign out a Coors Light. Even though we were there to help patients, we weren't able to offer long-term solutions or rehabilitation when it came to addiction. I wouldn't gain exposure to actually treating addiction until I was in nurse practitioner (NP) school, but these early experiences helped build my foundation as someone who wanted to do more than the bare minimum for these patients. I wanted to offer tangible, long-term support.

As I studied during NP school, I worked under a physician with a family practice. I treated patients of all ages with all sorts of ailments, and in doing so, I learned antibiotic dosages and chronic care management. I was also working with my first addiction patients. Part of this physician's practice involved medication-assisted treatment (MAT) for substance use disorders. Specifically, he prescribed Suboxone to those with opioid use disorder (OUD). I noticed a pattern during their initial visits: They were closed off, and they would look down at the floor when speaking to me. I could see that they were scared and embarrassed, beating themselves up.

Throughout their treatment, however, I would see something amazing happen. It wouldn't take long for these patients to turn their lives around with the right medication and encouragement. I remember one of these patients in particular who was able to transform himself. He had begun treatment before I joined the practice, but soon, I saw him standing tall with a spark in his eyes. He would smile and give me a hug, and we formed a strong relationship while at the clinic. I remember distinctly how excited he was to go back to school and how proud he was of his accomplishments—and I was proud of him too! I was invested in his recovery, as well as all the other patients with substance use disorders. These patients came to the clinic because they knew they had a problem and *wanted* help. I felt connected to them because I was also deeply invested in self-improvement, and this connection was reciprocated: Soon enough, the addiction patients seeking help were coming into the office, and the first question they would ask was, "Where's Trent?"

When we moved my family from Texas to my wife's hometown of Roswell, New Mexico, I saw intimately the reality of being afflicted with addiction and why these patients needed help. At the time, I was practicing as a nurse practitioner, making house calls for patients across the city. Although I wasn't there to treat addiction or substance use, I was exposed to the quality of life of an addict when there wasn't anyone around to help them. For some patients, their homes were in disrepair and unclean because they were struggling to get their lives on track. A few would speak openly to me and explain that they knew they had an issue but didn't know what to do or who to reach out to. I began looking into the resources available in the state of New Mexico and found out that the region was severely underserved. Even in larger cities like Las Cruces and Albuquerque, there were few easily accessible programs. It slowly dawned on me that this was how I could help the people who wanted help—the people I had gravitated toward throughout my entire career in healthcare. I realized that I needed to build the infrastructure for this underserved population—not only in New Mexico but hopefully, someday, across the rest of the country.

With this realization, I founded Renew Health. I jumped headfirst into the world of offering addiction recovery services, both in our brick-and-mortar clinics as well as telehealth services. When Renew Health first opened, I was still doing contract work as a nurse practitioner, but I was also doing as much outreach as I possibly could. I met with Rotary Clubs, other clinics and doctors, the CEOs of local hospitals and inpatient rehabilitation centers, and even the mayor of Roswell to educate everyone on what I was doing and gather information on how to best serve the community. It took six weeks to get my first patient through my door. She would also become my first success story. I've gone on to help thousands of patients overcome their addictions to substances, including alcohol, opioids, and methamphetamine, and I want to be able to do the same for anyone reading this book. Outpatient addiction treatment offers independence for patients, but it comes with its own challenges.

When a patient makes an appointment with us at Renew Health, and I have my first meeting with them, I recognize that this first appointment isn't the first step for them—they've already taken huge steps to acknowledge something needs to change in their lives, and they were brave enough to make an appointment and come in. As soon as they walk out the door, they will be confronted by barriers, triggers, and tests, which is a different experience from those who choose inpatient treatment. But that's why I try to be more than just somebody who prescribes solutions. I offer support and accountability for my patients so that they are able to be successful while recovering in reality—whether that be maintaining a job, raising their family, going to school, or whatever daily challenges present themselves outside of a clinic or treatment center.

The recovery journey is a deeply personal experience, unique to each individual's circumstances. It progresses from the trials of substance abuse toward the goal of sustained abstinence, but the path in between can vary greatly. For some, their greatest struggle may be during their initial detox. For others, it may be the maintenance of their sobriety despite life's stressors. Stopping substance use is the priority, but true recovery comes from transitioning to a healthier lifestyle with a trustworthy, sustainable support system. My job is to be a foundational pillar in that support system.

When I first meet patients, it's common for them to ask me about my own history with drug and substance use. I tell them that I'll occasionally have a drink or a cigar on the weekends, but I've never done any illicit drugs—I've never struggled with addiction personally, and some folks don't like to hear that. They may be looking for someone to make that connection with—someone who knows exactly what they're going through. Often, I have to explain: I've never struggled with addiction myself, and I don't have a family member or a close friend who's gone through it. I didn't come to this line of work because of a life-altering experience with addiction that made me realize this was my calling. I tell patients, "I'm here today doing this work because I want to be. I'm passionate about this. I'm interested in the medicine and recovery process. And I want to help you."

I started this work because I'm passionate about giving help to people who want help, but I continue this work because I have plunged into every avenue of addiction support and know that what I've learned will change lives. I want to use this book to break down stigma and inform readers that anyone with addiction can make their life better with the right tools and support. As you read, respond to what resonates with you. Not all of this may apply to your situation, but if you walk away with just a small amount of new knowledge, it may save you or the life of someone you love. If you, a friend, or a family member suffers from addiction, I want you to know that you are never down for the count, and I want to educate you on how you can do something about it. Recovery takes time, but with the right knowledge and help, anyone can rebuild their life. Why not you?

Throughout this book, I'll be addressing all the various tools you can pick up during your recovery. Each tool is unique in its application, but they all allow you to build up a strong and durable recovery. You'll even be surprised by what tools you're already familiar with. At the end of each chapter, you'll find a "workbench" where you can further familiarize yourself with the concepts and practice constructing a recovery that is all your own. By practicing with these tools, you'll gain the confidence to fill all the loops and pockets on your recovery tool belt and be on your way to living a fulfilling, sober life.

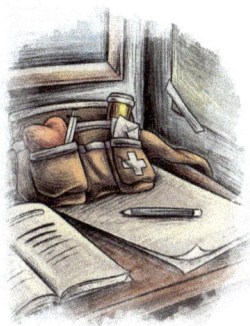

RECOVERY
WORKBENCH

Journal Prompts:

[?] What is your relationship with your addictive substance?

[?] What are your goals for recovery?

[?] Who are you now, and who do you want to become?

MAKE THIS BOOK YOUR OWN

By starting this book, you're already making a commitment to yourself and a commitment to your new life in recovery. Sometimes, it helps people to see this commitment put into words and sign an agreement as a way to officially start their journey.

Because of this, I have included a "Commitment to Self." Feel free to put pen to paper and sign this agreement if you think it will help your mindset going forward. You might be happy to discover how helpful it can be. Similarly, throughout this book, you're encouraged to highlight, underline, and mark up all the sections that resonate with you. Please write in the margins and, in response to the workbench sections, right there on the page. This is *your* tool belt, so while reading, don't be afraid to leave your mark.

COMMITMENT TO SELF:
A Personal Recovery Agreement

I, _____, am dedicated to living a life of health, healing, and freedom from addiction. My recovery is an ongoing process that requires my active participation and commitment. Through this agreement, I pledge to hold myself to the following promises:

- I commit to being an active participant in my recovery journey. I will take responsibility for my progress by showing up for myself each day, striving to make healthy choices, and seeking support when I need it.

- I pledge to attend all appointments with my treatment provider, including appointments for medication-assisted treatment or any other form of care I am receiving. I understand that my provider has my best interests at heart, and I will respect their guidance by adhering to the treatment plan we have agreed upon. If adjustments are needed, I will openly discuss them with my provider.

- I promise to be open and honest with my healthcare provider, counselors, and others involved in my recovery. I understand that honest communication is essential to building trust and ensuring that I receive the best care possible.

- I pledge to explore and make use of all resources available to me. This includes local health services, community centers, support groups, recovery programs, or any other resources that could help me build a strong foundation for an addiction-free life.

- I commit to educating myself about addiction, recovery, and the tools available to support my healing. I will make an effort to continue learning about my condition and how to maintain my sobriety long term.

I reaffirm my commitment to my recovery and my own well-being. I understand that my recovery is my responsibility, and by signing this agreement, I take full ownership of my journey. I acknowledge that setbacks may occur, but I pledge to keep moving forward and to never give up on myself.

I am worthy of a life free from addiction, and today, I commit to living that life.

Signature: _____

Date: _____

CHAPTER 1
TOOLS

- ☑ Addiction is a chronic medical disease influenced by neural patterns, genetics, environmental factors, and personal experiences, all of which can lead to harmful behavior. While it may feel like an intimidating task, addiction can be treated.

- ☑ Addictive substances drastically elevate dopamine levels far beyond natural highs, but over time, the body adapts by lowering the dopamine response, leading to tolerance, dependence, and a reduced ability to enjoy ordinary pleasures.

- ☑ A dependence is a physical need for a substance without compulsive behaviors, while an addiction includes harmful behavior despite negative consequences.

- ☑ Addiction can happen to anyone and does not discriminate.

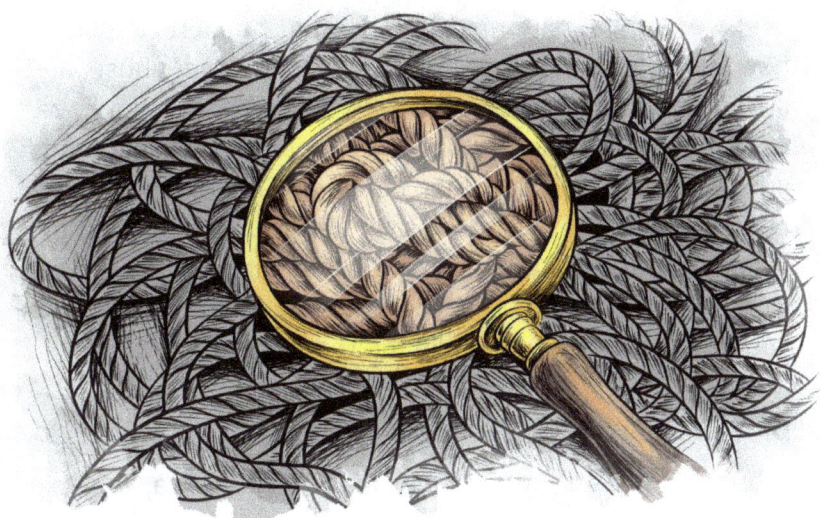

CHAPTER 1
OVERVIEW OF ADDICTION

When you're grappling with substance use disorder and addiction, you may feel like you're alone in your experience—like no one has experienced exactly what you're going through. But while your experience may be unique to you, there are plenty of people in the United States and around the world who have stories very similar to yours. According to a poll in 2023, two-thirds of Americans reported that "they or a family member have been addicted to alcohol or drugs, experienced homelessness due to addiction, or experienced a drug overdose leading to an emergency room visit, hospitalization, or death."[1]

Over the years, there have been fluctuations in usage, new substances that have risen to the forefront of abuse, and shifting opinions on addiction as a whole. There has never been a better time in history to get help with addiction and substance use disorders than right now. One of the ways we can help promote this idea is by better understanding the history and science of substance abuse in the United States. With the right knowledge and understanding of addiction, you or a loved one can begin the recovery journey.

BRIEF HISTORY OF SUBSTANCE ABUSE

When it comes to substance abuse in America, the "big three" are opioids, methamphetamine, and alcohol.

From a historical standpoint, opiate abuse in the US largely started during the Civil War with the introduction of morphine. Medics at that time would give soldiers this drug as medication after they received traumatic war injuries and mutilations. After the war, it continued to be abused by many. Along with morphine, opium was also used by those treating minor ailments such as headaches. The Bayer Company was actually the first company to introduce heroin back in 1898. Of course, they didn't understand its addictive qualities, and it was later pulled off of the shelves, but the damage was done, and it was soon being abused illegally. Even with the introduction and early evolution of these opiates, the abuse of opiates and opioids would not enter the mainstream until the 1990s.[2]

The modern opioid crisis in the United States began with a national pain advocacy campaign and the misleading marketing of newly reformulated opioid prescriptions.[3] Purdue Pharma introduced OxyContin in 1996 and touted that the drug had a 1 percent addiction rate. The reality was that this 1 percent addiction rate applied to patients receiving the drug in a hospital under regimented care, not to those prescribed it for self-administration.[4] What started as a seemingly great feat of marketing ended with thousands of people overdosing and dying. In 2007, Purdue was fined $600 million, and eventually, other opioid producers were sued for their misleading and life-altering tactics to sell more pills.[5] As a result of a crackdown on opioids, there was a resurgence of heroin and non-prescription opiates. In the 2010s, fentanyl became highly popularized because of its high potency and the ease of both manufacturing it and shipping it across the country.[6] Fentanyl is the cause of the worst addiction and overdose epidemic in the history of America, and it's where we find ourselves today. In 2021, the US surpassed 100,000 overdose deaths in a single year as a result of the fentanyl epidemic.[7]

Fentanyl was introduced fairly recently. In fact, when I was still working in the ICU, we often gave patients fentanyl to help them with pain. As a painkiller, it's extremely potent and effective when used appropriately. It's imperative to understand that it can only ever be safe at high doses when administered in a controlled setting: The patient is hooked up to monitors so that the medical professionals can check their respiratory rate, blood pressure, and every other life-ensuring measure. When fentanyl was introduced on the streets, it became drastically more popular, and we saw an increase in abuse. Other labels of opioids include hydrocodone, oxycodone, and numerous others—all "downers" created to help people with their pain.

Many people might not know the distinction between opiates and opioids. Opiates, including opium and morphine, are natural chemical compounds that have been extracted from poppy plants. Opioids, such as fentanyl or hydrocodone, have been either partially or completely synthesized in a laboratory. No matter their origin, they are both incredibly dangerous and addictive when abused or not taken under the supervision of a medical provider.

Opiates	Opioids
■ Opium ■ Morphine ■ Codeine ■ Thebaine	■ Fentanyl ■ Heroin ■ Hydrocodone ■ Oxycodone ■ Oxymorphone ■ Methadone ■ Meperidine

Methamphetamine, on the other hand, is a stimulant, or "upper." In 1932, it was first introduced in the US over the counter by the company Smith, Kline & French as a way to treat asthma and nasal congestion. Later, methamphetamine was manufactured to combat narcolepsy. During World War II, it was reported that soldiers from Japan, Germany, Britain, and the US used the stimulant during long military campaigns. Although the US tried to crack down on meth use in the 1980s, use of the stimulant skyrocketed in the '90s. "Between 1994 and 2004, methamphetamine use rose from just under two percent of the US adult population to approximately five percent." Meth use has decreased in the last decade, though Adderall and Ritalin, prescription medications used to treat ADHD that have similar properties to methamphetamine, are still widely prescribed and used in the US. Although they are considered a safer option, these drugs can still lead to addiction if they are mismanaged.[8]

Another common stimulant, cocaine, was first used as an anesthetic in the 1860s. Pharmaceutical companies began marketing the drug, although overdose deaths began to soar when cocaine was used during surgery. The use of cocaine in everyday life skyrocketed again when Coca-Cola added syrup to the drug and sold it as a tonic. It wasn't until 1903 that the company removed cocaine from the soda recipe. In the 1980s, another evolution of the drug, crack cocaine, caused cocaine usage to rise to 5.8 million people in the US.[9] Today, it is estimated that "27,788,000 US residents aged 12 and older used a form of cocaine at least once in their lifetime."[10]

Since opioids are downers, a lot of people who have an opioid addiction use a stimulant as a pick-me-up or as a way to get through an opioid withdrawal. This is an example of what happens when addicts use one drug to help with the symptoms of another drug, and it applies both ways. If someone is on methamphetamine, and they haven't slept in several days because of it, they might take fentanyl as a way to fall asleep. It creates a vicious cycle of abuse with detrimental effects.

As for the final component of the big three, alcohol has been around since the earliest civilizations of man, and, apart from Prohibition (1919–1933), alcohol has always been legal in the US.[11] It can be found at gas stations, grocery stores, and restaurants across the country. Because of this, it is the easiest substance to become addicted to from a societal acceptance standpoint. In 2022, 29.5 million people in the US, ages 12 and older, suffered from alcohol use disorder.[12] It was also estimated that 1 in 8 deaths among adults aged 20 to 64 were attributable to excessive alcohol.[13] Alcohol doesn't have the same stigma that some narcotics have, but it impacts millions of lives nonetheless.

THE SCIENCE OF ADDICTION

When you get down to it, the science behind these substances is all about the dopamine release. There's nothing we can organically do to our bodies that will match the feeling of elation that is fabricated by these substances. One strong drug can surpass something that you've worked a year for, like running a marathon. Typically, humans measure dopamine levels with a baseline of 100 that either increases or decreases depending on activity. For example, eating your favorite meal will bring your dopamine level to 150, and having sex will increase it to 200. The effect of substances on dopamine levels blow these numbers out of the water. Cocaine raises your dopamine level to 350, prescription opioids to 500, heroin to 900, and methamphetamine raises a normal dopamine level all the way up to 1,200.

Although these numbers stay steady when someone first takes a drug, over time, the high starts to decrease because of desensitization, and then, the baseline starts to decrease as well. So, while at first heroin can bring someone to 900, it slowly decreases and decreases to levels well below 800, which causes people to feel like they need to do more and more of the drug. And although someone's baseline used to be 100, it can decrease to 30 or 40—a level that makes it extremely hard to function or do simple tasks.[14] At these levels, if someone used to get a small dopamine spike from drinking coffee or seeing an old friend, those feelings are now exponentially minimized and would become extremely difficult to enjoy.

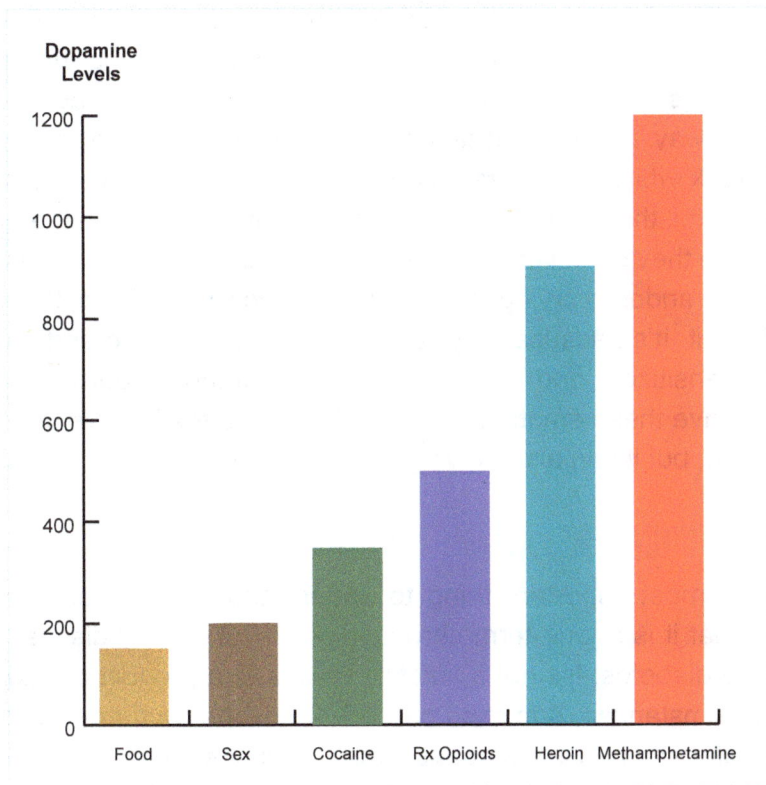

Dopamine Levels

Food	Sex	Cocaine	Rx Opioids	Heroin	Methamphetamine

Abusable substances, such as opiates and amphetamines, raise dopamine levels significantly higher than natural reinforcers.

The need to increase the dosage of the drug is also related to a defense mechanism in the body. Drug and alcohol tolerance develops as the body's defense mechanism against repeated exposure. Essentially, when a person regularly consumes drugs or alcohol, the body adapts to minimize the substances' effects and maintain balance in their internal environment. As a result, the individual needs to consume more of the substance to achieve the same effects. This process is the body's way of protecting itself from the potentially harmful effects of high levels of intoxicants.[15]

The flip side is that, once someone who uses these substances stops using them, they will start getting those feelings back. They can have all of these emotions again, in a way that can, at times, be overwhelming. If tragedy struck while they were still on drugs, and they never fully grieved, those feelings can all come crashing down on them when they get off of those drugs. I've seen patients who will start randomly crying, and they don't know why. Often, they hate it. It's because they've been numb for so long and so desensitized, and now their body is starting to learn how to have these emotions again. I think it's a really incredible thing, but it can also be very challenging up front.

DEBUNKING THE STIGMAS

The most important thing to understand about addiction is that it is a long-term chronic disease, like heart disease and diabetes. It's not a lifestyle choice or a product of bad circumstances. Addiction can affect anyone from any walk of life, and healing is not as simple as just stopping.

Another essential aspect to understand is that many people who think they are addicts actually just have a dependence. Often, someone will come into Renew Health and say they're an addict because their wife or co-worker told them that they were. For this specific reason, I have the American Society of Addiction Medicine's definition of addiction hung up on the wall: "Addiction is a treatable, chronic medical disease involving complex interactions among brain circuits, genetics, the environment, and an individual's life experiences. People with addiction use substances or engage in behaviors that become compulsive and often continue despite harmful consequences."[16] When I'm with a patient, I like to focus on the second sentence regarding behaviors. Oftentimes, patients who don't partake in compulsive and harmful behaviors are not addicts, they're just people with a physical or psychological dependence on a substance. They may never have abused a substance. Instead, maybe they were prescribed opioids after a traumatic car accident years ago, and they took the medication exactly as their doctor instructed, but if they were to stop taking that prescription, they would feel terrible and go into immediate withdrawal. This is a physical dependence. Patients will often come into the office with their heads down, feeling ashamed, and thinking their condition is so much worse than it actually is because of what people have been telling them. In this situation, it can be comforting when I, as a medical expert, tell them, "You're not an addict. Something really unfortunate happened to you, and now you're in this situation, but I don't see you as an addict."

So many people are just in pain and form a dependence. That's the nature of the beast, especially with opioids. When someone starts taking opioids, they are going to build a tolerance, and then they will need more and more. This cycle will continue, requiring the person to take a large amount of a substance for pain management, until they form an extreme physical dependence. This is not an addiction—the addictive behavior is not present.

On the other hand, when someone comes into the office who engages in addictive and harmful behaviors due to their reliance on substances, I can focus immediately on helping them in recovery. When it comes to what these specific behaviors are, some examples are lying, cheating, sneaking around, and stealing, all to support their condition. These are the behaviors that include paying for their addiction rather than paying for their water bill or going behind their spouse's back even after promising time and time again that they were done with substance abuse. It's a way of life that is continuous and detrimental to their well-being and the well-being of those around them. Whether someone's an addict or has a dependency, there's a wide spectrum of people who have a reliance on substances, and I know that I have the expertise and tools to help them, no matter where on the spectrum they may fall.

Unfortunately, some people are at a higher risk of developing an addiction or dependence than others. Geneticists have found evidence that certain people have a predisposition to drug and alcohol addiction. In fact, "genes are thought to account for about half of a person's risk of addiction." Scientists have even found certain genes that can help determine whether or not someone is predisposed to alcoholism.[17] That's not to say that someone will definitely become an addict if they are genetically predisposed, but if all the circumstances are stacked against them, some people have a higher likelihood of going down that path than someone else with the same external surroundings.

Something I found out extremely quickly when getting into this field is that addiction does not discriminate. In one day at Renew Health, I see so many different walks of life. Height doesn't matter. Sex doesn't matter. Race doesn't matter. Socioeconomic status doesn't matter. Occupation doesn't matter. There are so many people struggling with addiction, some of whom the outside world would never guess.

I had a patient once who was a young business professional taking care of his family. He had never touched a single drug in his life. One day, while walking into his carport, he slipped on his son's skateboard, causing him to fall and hit his back on the concrete steps. After five back surgeries and eight years of being in constant pain, he developed a dependence on opioids. He didn't do anything wrong—he was just trying to get to his car in the morning and didn't see his son's skateboard. He was in pain, and he medicated that pain with the best thing that was available to him at the time.

Another patient came into my office with a huge Louis Vuitton purse, Gucci shoes, Tom Ford glasses, and an expensive suit. She was a successful attorney who came from a very wealthy family, but she needed help. On the other side of the spectrum, we have unhoused members of the community who come in needing the exact same type of help as that attorney.

I've even met people outside of my practice who are addicted or dependent and don't show any outside indication of that being the case. When I was studying as a nurse practitioner, I met an attorney who took Adderall.

As someone who always digs for knowledge, I asked him, "Why are you taking Adderall? You're a practicing attorney and, obviously, very successful. Why?"

He responded, "Adderall gives me that edge. I can function so much higher with this stuff, so I take it."

I was fascinated and floored by this. He didn't have any reservations telling me about his Adderall abuse. Here was this extremely successful attorney who was abusing medication and probably didn't even know the severity of it at the time, all to give himself a competitive edge.

Once people realize they have a dependence or an addiction, there is a general lack of knowledge about the fact that treatments are even *available*, let alone that they actually work. This is because talking about addiction tends to be taboo in society. Even mainstream treatments, like methadone, are perceived as negative or scary. I think scary is the most prevalent word when discussing why more people don't know about treatment options because seeking help is *scary*. Even I, as a nurse practitioner, still get skittish about going to the doctor's office. There's something terrifying about facing the fact that there's an issue, having to be vulnerable, and having to share that with someone. And then, once you do talk to someone, there's a fear of hearing something you don't want to hear. In general, being at someone else's mercy and admitting there's a problem—especially for folks who have gone through withdrawal in the past, which is just about all of them—is a hard mountain to climb, but it's just the first step. So, in my personal practice, I try to make them feel as comfortable as possible because I know how scary it can be. This is all about making the patient feel heard and making them feel human.

Shame is a prevalent roadblock before seeking help. Sometimes, somebody can't even look me in the eyes. A lot of these people have their own biases about treatment, thinking that it will never work for them. So many patients have come into my office doubtful that their lives can change in an instant when they first reach out for help, but the most important stigma for me to debunk is that it *can* change that fast.

I have a new patient I've been seeing for three weeks who's a young guy in his 20s. He's got a daughter, he's not with her mom anymore, and he is so ashamed of his addiction. He wants to be a good father.

When he first came in, he had his elbows on his knees and was looking down. He started trying to talk, and then the tears came to his eyes.

He said, "Man, I want to do good. I want to be there for my daughter. I want to be a good parent. I'm doing it for me. I'm doing it for her. And I want to be there. I want to be a good role model and be a supportive father."

He summed up everything that a man wants to do for his daughter. So I got him on a treatment plan. And lo and behold, one week later, he's looking better, feeling better, and not breaking into tears. He was just smiling and looking me in the eye. All these things happened in one week.

It was so clear to me that he just wanted to be a good dad. He told me all these things he and his daughter did during the week: running around town, going to the park, and having a blast. And his daughter couldn't believe it because her daddy was playing with her. She loved that he was being fun and that he wasn't angry or upset at himself. That's one of the greatest patient stories for me. Being a father myself and having a daughter who also loves when I support her and do fun things with her, it gave me the most profound joy to help another man be there for his daughter.

This patient loves when I give him high fives. And I love making him feel supported and built up. As a result, he can't wait to come back for his next visit and continue his treatment because he feels so good.

Whether it's a high five or a hug or just a good, firm handshake, I try to congratulate all my patients because I know how many hurdles they had to overcome to get to my office and do the work.

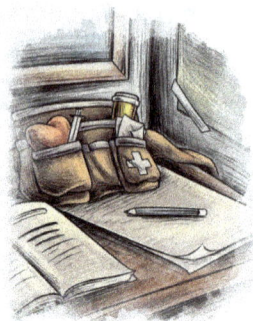

RECOVERY
WORKBENCH

Journal Prompts:

[?] Have you or a loved one ever felt stigmatized by others?

- How did it make you feel?
- How did you react?

[?] What's something you wish you could help others understand about substance abuse or your own personal experience with it?

[?] What is something you've learned about addiction that has surprised you?

[?] What's something you used to enjoy before your addiction that you hope to be able to enjoy again while in recovery?

TOOLS

☑ Honesty and transparency are required when working with healthcare professionals as that information allows for a personally effective treatment plan.

☑ Family and friends should understand addiction is a chronic disease and should be treated as such. It is not a moral failure.

☑ A support network can extend beyond friends and family into support groups, counselors, and former addicts.

☑ Limit interactions with people who enable substance use and build a network that supports your recovery journey.

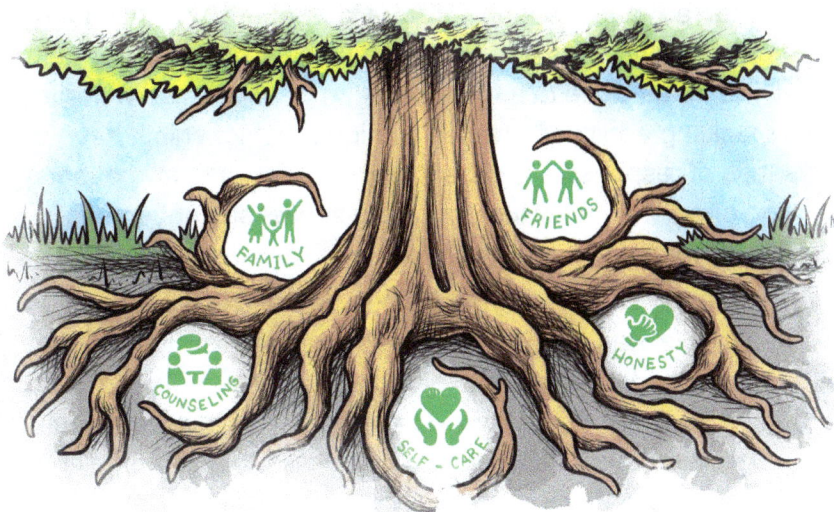

CHAPTER 2
A FOUNDATION
OF SUPPORT

One of the most challenging aspects of the recovery process is undoubtedly taking that first step: acknowledging there's a problem. It requires immense courage to admit that, not just to oneself, but also in front of others. Once that barrier is crossed, openly discussing the problem often brings its own set of challenges, as it tends to involve confronting painful realities and vulnerabilities. At Renew Health, we do our best to create a foundation of trust and care that all patients can come to rely on. This foundation is necessary for everyone's recovery journey.

For anyone walking through our doors, I'm not their friend—I'm first and foremost a healthcare professional. But I try to be as close to a friend as I can be. The trust we forge by tackling addiction creates a unique relationship. I have a sense of responsibility to be there for the care of my patients wholeheartedly. In return, my most successful patients take their recovery very seriously.

Anthony was pretty young when he first came into Renew Health. He was in his early 20s, depressed, struggled with fentanyl and alcohol, out of work, and his girlfriend had left him. When I first met him, Anthony had a hard time maintaining eye contact with me. He was thinking of taking his own life and was incredibly scared. Even still, he was receptive to the treatment plan I shared with him. When leaving the office, he felt a little skeptical, but also optimistic.

Once he was on medication and under our care, he had an immediate turnaround. By week one, I could see him improving. By week two, he looked physically healthier. His life just took off from there. He got a job. He was no longer suicidal, and his depression subsided. After about six months, we were even meeting over video calls through telehealth services rather than meeting in person. Everything was going great until one day when I was running late to our call.

I was five minutes late, finishing up with a patient, when my receptionist received a phone call from Anthony.

"Where's Trent?" he asked, brashly.

My receptionist clocked this as odd behavior as Anthony usually has much more patience and understanding.

"He's finishing up with a prior patient, but he'll be right with you," she replied.

"Well, tell him to hurry up," said Anthony.

When this got back to me, I could tell something was wrong. I got on the video call, and I could see Anthony pacing around his room. The phone's camera was shaking in his hand.

Anthony said, "Doc, I relapsed."

I said, "That's alright. Here's what we'll do—"

"*Man*, I got drunk. I beat the shit out of a cop. I'm on the run. They're coming after me!"

"Oh."

I was shocked: Anthony had made his appointment on time and was mad at me for being late, all while he was on the run from the cops. Anthony explained how he got drunk, and the cops were called. He hit one of the cops and ran away. I told him immediately, "Dude, you need to turn yourself in. This is not gonna go good for you."

Anthony spiraled out of control.

"I'm gonna go to prison, and you're not gonna be able to take care of me anymore," he cried.

I assured Anthony that I'd still be his provider and make sure he got his medication wherever he needed it to be sent, but that right now, he needed to turn himself in.

Anthony did turn himself in, and I saw him back in the office a couple months later. He's back in treatment. But that experience reminded me of the bond I have with my patients. Anthony was dedicated to his recovery journey, even if that meant calling into a video call while on the run from the cops. That was dedication in its most extreme form, but I see it with all my patients who are working hard to better themselves.

I'll always be in their corner, even when they slip up. Lapses, relapses, mistakes—they happen. We're all human. But when my patients slip up, they often feel like they're letting me down personally. I have one patient who lapsed and later told me that while he was taking drugs, he was thinking, "Dammit, Trent's gonna be mad at me." I wasn't mad, but I'm glad that my motivation is taken to heart by my patients.

At Renew Health, I always try to instill in my patients that, no matter the phase of their recovery journey, they are never alone. It's what I wish I could say to everyone struggling with addiction. When seeking a healthcare provider, finding someone who will always be in your corner can be a huge advantage when you begin recovery. Building that kind of relationship can take time, but it's worth it in the end.

THE INTERVIEWS

When a new patient first comes in, our initial meeting is pivotal. Right from the start, they come to me looking for answers. They understand they have a problem, and they need to trust that I will be able to give them solutions. Most of the time, I have the power of modern medicine to offer up as the best course of action, but I need more than that to curb their addiction. I need to create an environment where they feel comfortable enough to share detailed and personal stories without fear of judgment. Patients trust me to listen to and validate their experiences. Once I learn about a patient, we can collaborate and design a treatment plan that addresses their specific needs. I work hard to give my patients my full attention, without interruptions. They should know that my time with them is *their* time—I genuinely want to hear what they have to say and show them the respect they deserve. I also try to be mindful of my body language by maintaining eye contact and sitting in a relaxed, open manner. No matter what they share with me, I never want to come across as uncomfortable or shocked. This first encounter is about laying a foundation of trust and understanding, ensuring they know they're heard and truly understood.

I call these initial meetings "interviews" not only because I'm interviewing the patients, but because they're interviewing me. I'm trying to get as much information as I can from a patient so I know *how* to help them, but they're surveying me to see if I even *can* help them. It's my job to inform them, show that I have the best solution for them, and build trust as immediately and honestly as I can. I start by letting them know that everything we talk about is confidential, meaning they can share anything they want with me, and that information stays between us. So if a judge comes and knocks on my door, I legally don't have to give them anything. All stories shared in this book are only added with explicit consent from the patient. Also, many of the substances that patients use are illicit, which may cause them to feel uncomfortable sharing more about their condition. There's no judgment from me; if I can make that clear, I will have more honest interactions with them, which makes it easier to help them.

When I'm listening to a patient for the first time, I'm not just hearing their words; I'm paying attention to a few key things. I try to pick up on underlying emotions that might not be immediately obvious. Sometimes, it's in the tone of their voice, their body language, or even what they're not saying. I also listen closely to their personal history and any patterns that come up. Knowing their past experiences, what's worked or hasn't worked for them, and any triggers they have helps me tailor the treatment plan to fit their unique needs. Another thing I focus on is their motivation and readiness to change. This helps me figure out the best approach to support them and keep them motivated. I'm also on the lookout for any immediate risks, like signs of severe depression or thoughts of self-harm so that we can address those right away.

Honesty and transparency are absolutely crucial in this process. When a patient is open with me, it allows me to get the full picture of what they're going through. This means I can address the real issues at hand more effectively. If they hold back or aren't completely honest, we might miss critical pieces of the puzzle, which can hinder their progress. It's also true that, sometimes, we don't have time to go into the full picture or discuss the treatment plan when we first meet. If a patient is in the midst of withdrawal, they're so uncomfortable that my immediate priority is providing relief.

Not long ago, I walked into one of our rooms to meet with a new patient and her mom, only to find the young woman laying on her stomach, face in the carpet, arms and legs splayed out like a starfish. I looked at the mother and asked, "What's going on here?"

"She's in severe withdrawal," said the mom.

From the ground, the young woman let out a single groan and muttered, "Miserable."

That became a very quick first visit. I got the information I needed, prescribed Suboxone, and sent them directly to the pharmacy. I ended up meeting with her the following week, and she was a completely different person. She was over the withdrawal, smiling, and ready to tell me more about herself. From there, we discussed the long-term goals of her treatment plan.

I'll meet with patients more frequently in the first few months of their treatment. With medication-assisted treatment, there's a balance of trying doses and matching them to your symptoms. Some doctors have a patient come in and want to diagnose them in the first 20 seconds. I never want to make any assumptions with patients; that is what leads to misdiagnosis. If a patient is upfront about their struggles, whether it's a relapse or a tough emotional spot, we can address it right away and adjust the treatment plan accordingly. As a treatment provider, it's my responsibility to ensure they get the best support possible for their recovery. I'm not the only one supporting them though—my Renew Health team is also part of that foundation of care. The first time you meet with a new provider, remember to be open with them and to take the time to tell them your story. This will help *them* help *you*.

RENEW HEALTH AND YOUR FIRST STEPS

When someone looking for relief from addiction comes to Renew Health, I'm happy to be there for them, but it's not just my support they're getting. I have a whole team that helps run our office, our services, and maintains the important cornerstones of trust, motivation, and care.

Building the right team is crucial to our success. I look for loyalty, ambition, and drive in individuals, but it starts with a fundamental connection—I need to like them. Compatibility and a pleasant work environment are non-negotiable for me because they directly affect our ability to provide exceptional patient care. When my staff is friendly, and everyone enjoys their work, it creates a positive atmosphere that patients notice immediately. I believe this is essential for effective patient care, as a happy team naturally enhances the healing environment.

Plenty of first-time patients come in and are scared. Some will even sit in the waiting room, fill out all the forms provided to them, and then get up and leave. My staff are confident in their ability to help anyone who walks through the door and strive to make the environment as un-scary as possible. They've helped so many people already; they know that anyone with addiction or substance use disorder can find relief in our practice. For anyone who is uncertain about their recovery journey, we're patient and understanding.

Few people on my staff have personally struggled with substance abuse. However, many of them have dealt with other mental health challenges, such as anxiety and depression. Additionally, several of our team members have family members who have struggled with substance abuse, which gives them a deep understanding and empathy for the struggles our patients face. Their experiences help them connect with and support our patients in meaningful ways. Every member of our staff brings compassion and understanding to their roles. Even if it's just in the form of a bright smile for the people walking in, it's incredibly valuable to our work.

From the moment a patient walks through our doors, they should feel safe and respected. Our staff are trained to be approachable and supportive, making it clear that they're here to help, not judge. Patients need to know that anything they share with us stays between us. By consistently respecting their privacy and maintaining a safe space, we build a foundation of trust that allows patients to open up and fully engage in their recovery journey. Again, patients have already taken the first steps by admitting they have a problem and getting care. We want to make sure our team supports every single step once they come to us for help.

Every addiction clinic should prioritize hiring compassionate individuals. Each time someone walks into a clinic, they should be greeted with a genuine smile from someone who wants to help and someone who feels proud of the patient walking in. For all the support we can provide, patients also need to recognize and cultivate support from everyone else in their lives.

FINDING YOUR SUPPORT SYSTEM

Family and friends play a crucial role in the recovery process. They offer emotional support, practical help, and accountability, which can significantly enhance the chances of long-term success. While individuals without a strong support network can and do achieve recovery, the journey can be smoother and often more effective with supportive loved ones involved. These relationships provide encouragement during tough times, celebrate successes, and help maintain a stable environment conducive to recovery. The best way for a support network to start helping is to educate themselves on addiction.

An important lesson for anyone learning about substance use disorder: Addiction is a disease. Family and friends should understand that it's not a choice, a moral failure, or a lack of willpower—addiction is a disease that alters the brain and requires care and patience to overcome. This knowledge helps shift their perspective from blame to support, which is essential for creating a positive environment. I also emphasize the importance of patience and empathy. Recovery is an often long and challenging journey, and loved ones will need consistent support and understanding along the way. Even during setbacks like a relapse, it's important not to judge and instead offer words of encouragement. Attending therapy sessions, joining support groups, and educating themselves about addiction and recovery can make a huge difference. The more they know and understand, the better they can support their loved one effectively.

I had a patient who struggled with multiple relapses, but finally found stability when their family got involved. The family attended counseling sessions and learned how to provide the best support, which made a huge difference. I've also seen the power of spousal support. One of my patients was successful in their recovery because their spouse encouraged their treatment and even attended therapy sessions with them to rebuild their relationship. Having someone in your corner offers an immense amount of motivation. Whether it's a spouse, parent, sibling, or friend, I've seen how their encouragement and setting of healthy boundaries helped the patient develop the skills needed to stay sober. This renewed bond can easily become a cornerstone of their support system.

When loved ones understand the challenges and learn how to provide effective support, the entire recovery journey can be more supported and less isolating. Encouraging family therapy or support groups for friends and family can also be beneficial, as it helps them navigate their roles in the recovery process more effectively. Having someone in your corner, outside of your healthcare specialist team, goes a long way. Unfortunately, not everyone has access to a reliable support system.

One of my patients didn't have a reliable support network of family or friends who they could turn to during their recovery process. Because a support system is especially important during detox, this patient's only option in this case was inpatient detox at a facility, rather than our typical outpatient option at home where a support system can watch over the patient. Since there was a waitlist for inpatient detox, she had to go back to using drugs for a short period to mitigate withdrawal symptoms. This is a last resort and never ideal.

If you can't get support from friends or family, I always recommend finding a network elsewhere because having people who want to understand and can offer encouragement is imperative. One great option is joining a support group. There are plenty of groups out there, like Alcoholics Anonymous or Narcotics Anonymous, where people share their experiences and provide mutual support. It's a great way to connect with others who are going through similar challenges. I would also recommend searching for a therapist or counselor who specializes in addiction treatment. With their expertise, they can offer professional advice tailored to their patients' needs. Resources can be found on a community level as well, including recovery coaches or peer support specialists who can provide one-on-one support. Finding additional support can be as easy as going online. Online forums and social media groups are a valuable resource for anyone who may have difficulty meeting in person. No matter where a patient is, there are communities looking to support one another's recoveries. Outside of recovery-related groups, I encourage patients to get involved in activities or hobbies that interest them, which can be a great way to meet new people and build a supportive social network. Whether it's joining a sports team, taking a class, or volunteering, engaging in positive activities can provide a sense of community, ideally replacing the community who previously enabled your substance abuse.

Building a better community can feel difficult if everyone around you is also abusing substances. Another young patient of mine felt really isolated after she stopped using street drugs because many of her friends were still using. Then a childhood friend reconnected with her and introduced her to a new, supportive, and sober social circle. That new network played a crucial role in her recovery. It's extremely important for patients to create a safe and encouraging environment for their recovery, which sometimes means distancing themselves from friends or family who encourage substance use. To do this, it's crucial to set clear boundaries: Patients should communicate openly and firmly with those individuals, explaining their commitment to recovery and the need to avoid situations where substance use is present. It's okay to be honest and let them know that continuing the relationship as it was before isn't healthy. This might mean patients eventually need to find new social circles that support their sobriety.

Surrounding yourself with people who understand and support your journey can make a big difference. If it's difficult to avoid certain individuals completely, I suggest limiting interactions to safe, controlled environments where substance use is unlikely to occur. For example, meet at a coffee shop instead of a bar, or meet during the day rather than at night. It's important to have a plan in place for dealing with high-risk situations. This might include having a trusted friend to call for support, practicing what to say if offered drugs, and knowing when to leave if the situation becomes too tempting. I recommend patients be open and honest with their support system. Asking for help strengthens trust, but be careful not to become over-reliant on that support. The goal is to develop self-reliance—a trust in one's own abilities and limits. By setting boundaries, finding supportive social networks, and planning ahead, patients can protect their recovery and stay focused on their goals.

Self-care is important for everyone, so support systems need to take care of themselves as well. Supporting someone through recovery can be emotionally taxing, so it's vital that family and friends also prioritize their own mental and physical health. This ensures they can be there for their loved one without burning out. Burnout does happen. I've had patients use up every ounce of goodwill from their family and friends, leaving them with a strained relationship.

Kaylee's family had spent thousands of dollars for her to go to multiple inpatient rehabs across the country. They were nice, luxurious centers, and Kaylee was sober while she was there, but once she was out, she would immediately relapse. When Kaylee first came to see me, she was with her sister-in-law.

"I'm here to support Kaylee, but I don't think this is going to work. This is the last straw," said the sister-in-law.

When it came time for Kaylee to detox at home, she was terrified. She didn't want her parents or family to be around for that and was asking for a hotel room for the weekend.

To this request, the sister-in-law replied, "No, because you're going to have drugs there within 20 minutes after we do that. I know exactly what's going to happen."

Kaylee didn't come back the next week. And I didn't see her for a while, but eventually, she returned to Renew Health on her own accord. Her attitude was completely different. She told me she wanted to go back to work. She wanted to be with her kids again. She was tired of living with addiction. The support from her family was enough to keep her alive up to this point, but it was only when *she* wanted a life without addiction that her recovery journey meant more to her.

Addiction creates strains on relationships with parents, siblings, children, spouses, partners—*everyone*. You can get as much support as possible from your team, but if you aren't dedicated to your recovery, you'll just be burning bridges. When building a foundation of support during a recovery journey, be mindful of the work everyone is putting in and make the most of it.

The journey to recovery is unique for everyone. There's no one-size-fits-all approach; we're here to find what works best for our patients and anyone struggling with addiction. Taking the first step can be intimidating, but you're not alone. It's okay to feel nervous or uncertain. Recovery is a process that requires time, patience, and effort. There will be ups and downs, but every step forward, no matter how small, is progress. Patients want to build a healthier, happier future, and we're committed to helping our patients achieve that. Just by deciding to go to a clinic, you're already making a significant, positive change in your life. By laying the foundation of support, from your healthcare specialist to your family and friends, you can then look toward accomplishing your sobriety goals.

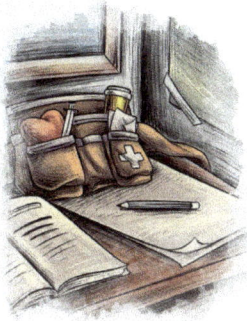

RECOVERY
WORKBENCH

Journal Prompts:

[?] What does taking the first step toward recovery mean to you?

- How does taking that first step feel, or how do you imagine it will feel?

[?] If your loved one has ever struggled with substance abuse, how did you show that you were there for them?

[?] What kind of support do you need from your support system?

- How can you let them know what you need from them?

[?] What do you look for in a healthcare professional in order to trust them?

- In what ways can you open up more during appointments so that you can build up that relationship?

CHAPTER 3
TOOLS

☑ A treatment plan should be developed together with a healthcare provider for long-term recovery.

☑ Goals are useful tools to measure success and set milestones toward future sobriety.

☑ Gathering knowledge on addiction and recovery, such as how medication works and how to manage side effects, allows patients to be active in their own recovery.

☑ Setbacks happen, but a lapse or relapse doesn't mean that sobriety isn't still possible.

☑ Detoxification and withdrawal can be a daunting and stressful experience. Consult with your healthcare professional to make sure you have a safe detox, especially with alcohol detox, which can be deadly.

☑ Financial resources and programs are available on a local, state, and national level to make sure that anyone who needs treatment can receive it.

☑ Telehealth is a viable option for recovery, allowing for remote support and treatment on your own schedule.

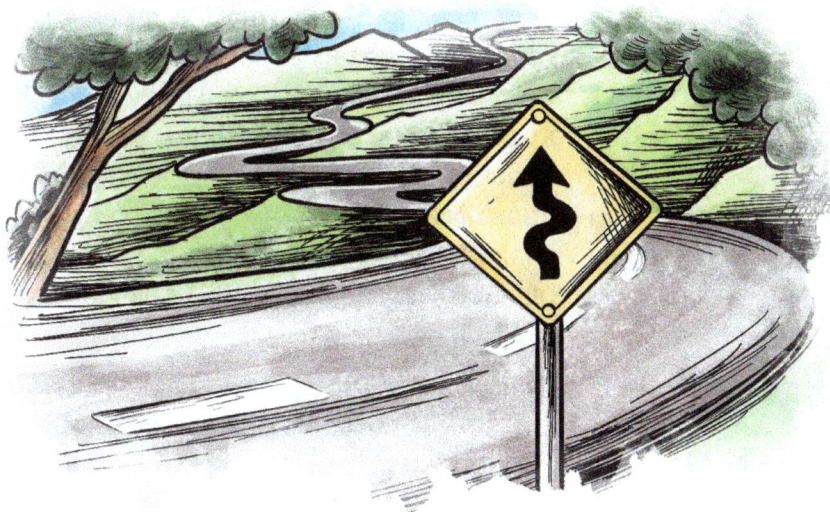

REALISTIC EXPECTATIONS

Many people who go to an addiction clinic for their first appointment aren't certain how their recovery journey will unfold. Whether they've been through withdrawal and recovery before or they're trying treatment for the first time, many patients usually have some unrealistic expectations that need to be addressed.

Sometimes, patients think they can skip detox and withdrawal. I always explain that it's an unavoidable step, but there are available medications that make withdrawal as comfortable as possible. Other times, patients have the expectation that they only need to be on addiction medication for a couple of weeks or months. I explain that this process is a marathon, not a sprint. We then talk about the history and timeline of their addiction. If it's been 12 years, I'll say, "Okay, so you have 12 years on that side of the scale, and you want to be off of the addiction medication after 6 months?" This helps to put it in perspective. Being on this medication isn't a bad thing. As I've said, addiction is a chronic illness. How do we treat chronic illnesses like heart disease or diabetes? With medication. And it takes time and work if you want to come off the medication.

Nothing in life worth having comes at the click of a button, and sobriety is no different. It won't happen overnight. Even if, one day, someone stops drinking or using drugs completely, it will continue to be an ongoing process—no one can just flip a switch between their ears. This is the case for everyone working on their health. If someone achieves a healthy lifestyle, it takes work every single day to maintain that. Also, this isn't just true of a healthy lifestyle. It extends to everything in life that's truly valuable: marriages, friendships, long-lasting careers, etc. If it's valuable, you can bet it will take time. This is something I make sure to be entirely upfront about with my patients so that when we start talking about their treatment and sobriety goals, they have a realistic expectation of what they're agreeing to.

GOAL SETTING

Once we've established a comfortable and trusting environment, my focus shifts to the practical steps of assessment, diagnosis, and developing a treatment plan. I take a thorough look at both their medical history and the concerns they bring to the table that day. Together, we tailor a treatment plan that not only addresses the immediate symptoms but also aims at long-term health and recovery. It's a collaborative effort where their input and my expertise come together to craft a path forward.

Goals are meant to be a North Star to guide a patient through their recovery. General goals, such as maintaining sobriety, establish a foundation for a patient's rehabilitation. Short-term goals, including taking medication as prescribed, participating in support groups, or attending regular therapy sessions, are what really define the recovery experience. Accomplishing these goals is what develops healthy daily routines. As we progress, the goals become more specific and can include timelines like building a new career, re-establishing relationships, and maintaining sobriety milestones like six months or a year.

When establishing goals with a patient, I consider their overall well-being and leave room to allow for adjustments as needed. I prefer talking to people casually so I can get right down to figuring out the best way to help them. A relaxed person-to-person connection opens patients up and allows them to share their wants and personal goals more easily. They can tell that I'm giving them support and that I have their best interests at heart. But at the same time, I'm specific about how I'm going to tailor their treatment to help them, how they'll start feeling better in a week, and, best of all, how it's entirely achievable. This approach is flexible because it's not so structured. It's human. The most important key to this is to make sure the patient feels empowered and supported throughout the process to keep them dedicated to their goals. When goals are achieved, we celebrate those wins and continuously reassess and adjust to ensure they're motivated and moving forward.

KNOWLEDGE IS POTENTIAL POWER

Early on in the recovery process, I like to make sure a patient understands that knowledge isn't power; rather, knowledge is *potential* power, meaning once I give a patient the knowledge, it's completely up to them to follow through. Taking action is the real power. Knowledge is a tool on the recovery tool belt that helps them take action and participate in their own sobriety. It's almost like a tape measure that allows a patient to know where to start drilling and hammering.

When patients have a clear understanding of their medication and treatment plan, their confidence levels noticeably increase. Knowing the "why" and "how" behind their treatment empowers them and gives them a sense of control over their recovery process. Because of this, I make it a point to thoroughly explain every aspect of their recovery plan, including how the medications work, what timelines they can expect, and how to manage any potential side effects. This transparency helps clarify the process and alleviates a lot of anxiety. When meeting with your provider, don't be afraid to ask questions if they don't explain something thoroughly.

The amount of information a patient needs depends on the person. Some people want to know everything in the first meeting, and then they come back a week later after doing their own research online and are now "Dr. Google." Other people are very experienced in the recovery process and simply need to know where to pick up their addiction medication because they already know the symptoms they will experience. For patients like this, I just need to give them the medications they need and continue to hold them accountable. Whatever level of information a person requires, I have several handouts and patient portals with troves of information that I make available to every patient who walks into Renew Health as well as anyone not in New Mexico who needs a place to start gathering information.

It's one thing to learn about addiction and recovery, but it's another to apply that knowledge in your daily life. This also means that any win you achieve is your win alone.

Recently, a man came to his first appointment with his wife as his support system. He was struggling with an alcohol addiction. While he went into the room for his appointment, his wife stayed in the lobby. When I saw her sitting there, she looked really sad and frustrated. I could tell their relationship had been put through the wringer because of his addiction. Every day, he was getting drunk at 7 a.m. and would stay drunk all day long. Although she was visibly frustrated with her husband, she obviously wasn't giving up on him and still very much loved him. The weight and guilt of that was written all over this patient's face and shown in his body language. He was ashamed.

One week later, after being on the medication, he said to me, "It worked. I haven't drank since that morning before our first appointment." He went on to say, "You did it. You did all this for me."

I responded, "I didn't do this. You did this. I just gave you some tools, but that's it. You figured out how to use those tools and dug yourself out of it."

Every week, I have patients who go through a holistic lifestyle change in an astonishingly short time. Often, they're very appreciative, so they want to thank me and tell me their success was due to my help. And every time this happens, I have to remind them that I just gave them a tool belt. They're the ones in control. They're the ones who came in, educated themselves, and took the medication. They pulled a tool off the belt, got to work, and built something new—a life beyond addiction.

I'm doing this work to help my patients, not to be thanked. But I would be lying if I said it doesn't feel good. It's amazing to see how much progress one person can make in a week. You'll be astonished to find this out for yourself on your own journey with your very own tool belt.

RECOVERY IS NOT A STRAIGHT LINE

When it comes to setting expectations, patients need to confront the reality of setbacks. I often describe recovery as driving on a highway—it's not always a straight or smooth journey. There are bumps along the way, and sometimes, it's okay to take an exit and find our way back onto the path a little down the road. The important thing is that we're continuously moving in the right direction, even if there are some closed roads, potholes, or traffic. No matter how small, every step forward is a victory in the recovery journey. Describing it this way provides a clear and relatable visual for patients to understand the different phases and challenges along the way. The goal is to keep progressing and not get discouraged by temporary setbacks.

It's imperative not to view these setbacks as failures, but rather as opportunities to learn and grow. By normalizing setbacks and discussing them openly, we take away some of the fear and shame that can come with them. This understanding allows patients to be more forgiving of themselves and enables them to stay committed to their recovery, even when things don't go perfectly. It's all about building resilience and focusing on long-term progress rather than short-term perfection.

Focusing on the positives is a great way to get through a setback. In these situations, I do my best to build patients up when they're being particularly hard on themselves. I remind them that they've gotten sober before, and they can do it again. There was one patient, Evan, who was struggling with an opioid addiction for six years. When he first started treatment with me, he was 13 days sober before he had a lapse. He was really putting himself down until I helped him put it into perspective.

I said to him, "Evan, it's been 6 years since you've been sober, and you just went 13 days without using. That's the biggest accomplishment you've had in almost a decade when it comes to this. That's amazing, man."

You have to celebrate the accomplishments, no matter how small they may seem to others. Then, it's about learning from what happened. I said to Evan, "You just went 13 days sober. You can do it again." Evan and I broke it down together: How did you do it? What system do we implement now to help you do it again? What kept you motivated during those 13 days? How did the medication feel? What triggered the lapse? It's through asking questions like these that we can turn a setback into an opportunity to establish long-term sobriety.

Whether someone lapsed back to a substance for a couple of days or completely relapsed back into their addiction, it can be incredibly upsetting and shouldn't be downplayed. But the nature of life is that everything valuable will be elusive at times. Focusing on the positives helps to ensure people can find their way back to the recovery highway.

I have found that a patient's intrinsic motivation is most effective in getting them back on that highway—almost like an internal recovery GPS. Some people come to Renew Health because their boss told them they would get fired if they didn't get sober, or their spouse told them they would divorce them if they didn't change. While this can be very motivating to get someone to the first appointment, long-term recovery doesn't happen until the motivation is also found within the patient.

Helping patients find their intrinsic motivation connects them to their deeper, personal reasons for wanting to recover. We start by having open, honest conversations about what truly matters to them. This could be their family, career aspirations, personal health, or dreams they want to achieve. To discover what truly matters to you, I encourage you to reflect on your values and envision a life without the burden of addiction. Visualize your future—what do you want it to look like? How do you want to feel? Try to see beyond the immediate struggles and focus on the bigger picture.

Envisioning a better future sometimes doesn't mean focusing on something big. It could mean focusing on something people often take for granted, like getting the water turned back on at your house so that your kids can shower from home. Once patients get something like that back, they're motivated to keep it, which helps them hold a steadier job, work on budgeting, and avoid wasting hundreds of dollars a week on drugs.

If someone doesn't find their internal motivation, they are usually the patient who comes in one time and then says, "Lose my number." Building up the necessary momentum requires catching people at the right time with the right motivation. Setting small, achievable goals that align with their intrinsic values and interests will often spark that inner drive to keep going. And that inner drive to keep going is imperative for certain points of the recovery process, most notably: detox.

THE REALITY OF DETOX

Detox is the first procedure of recovery. It's also normally the biggest deterrent.

Detox, or detoxification, is the process where the body clears itself of drugs or alcohol. It is challenging because the body is adjusting to functioning without the substance it's become dependent on. During detox, the body starts to rid itself of the toxins accumulated from substance use, which can trigger a variety of physical and psychological withdrawal symptoms, ranging from mild to severe. Physically, someone might experience symptoms like sweating, shaking, nausea, vomiting, muscle aches, and fatigue. Depending on the substance, there can also be more serious symptoms like seizures, heart palpitations, or death. Psychologically, detox can cause symptoms such as anxiety, depression, irritability, and intense cravings for the substance. The brain is essentially trying to rewire itself after becoming accustomed to the presence of the substance, which can lead to these emotional and mental challenges.[1]

It's very important to go through detox under medical supervision, especially for substances like alcohol and benzodiazepines, where withdrawal can be particularly dangerous—even lethal. Medical professionals can provide support and medications to help manage withdrawal symptoms and make the process as safe and comfortable as possible. Even for substances that are less dangerous, medically managed detox can lessen the severity and duration of withdrawal.

At Renew Health, we try to alleviate the fear around detox as much as possible. Providing thorough education about what to expect can reduce anxiety quite a bit. When you know what's coming, it's often less scary. I make sure to explain the detox process in detail, including the symptoms they might experience and how we can manage them. I also emphasize that they won't be going through it alone.

Choosing medically managed detox means that healthcare professionals will be available to support you with regular check-ins and address any discomfort or complications that arise. Knowing that a team is there to ensure your safety and well-being can be very reassuring. I also recommend relying on your support system during detox. Whether it's involving family, friends, or support groups, having a network of people who care can make a huge difference. Emotional support can help you feel less isolated and more confident in facing the challenge. And physical support is invaluable when it's difficult to even get out of bed.

Additionally, emotions that were previously suppressed by substance use tend to resurface during sobriety. This can be confusing and challenging, as you may experience intense emotions that seem unfamiliar or disproportionate to the current circumstances. Addressing these emotions through therapy, support groups, and healthy coping mechanisms is crucial to helping you navigate your feelings and build emotional resilience during and after detox.

Renew Health offers "at-home" detox, but inpatient detox is also an option. At an inpatient facility, the patient is under 24/7 supervision and is given fluids and medications through IVs. At home, a patient is able to have telehealth visits with us and is able to reach me at any time if questions arise. This is a great option, especially if family members are available to provide care and immediate treatment is needed. For inpatient facilities, there can sometimes be waiting lists and other restrictions, like insurance, that put someone's recovery on hold. When I schedule at-home detox with my patients, I work around their lives, even when it comes to ensuring they don't have to take any time off of work. With medically managed detox, we can plan for the worst of it to occur over the weekend. By anticipating the timeline of a patient's detox, the most severe symptoms can be experienced at the most convenient time for the patient.

The reality of detox is that even when someone has the help of medications or a facility, it will feel awful. Sometimes, it's the worst people have ever felt, especially if they try to white-knuckle it with no help. Many who choose this path don't even know there's a better, less painful option through medically managed detox. When this is the case with my patients, I always tell them, "Well, tell your friends that there's a better way and that they should come see me. I can help make their detox so much easier." There's a reason why practically all of my patients opt for medically managed detox when given the choice.

It's important to note that once a patient has detoxed, the danger of overdosing increases. This is because tolerance decreases after detox and sustained abstinence. If an individual relapses after an extended period of sobriety, they should use a much lower dose than when they were actively using. Relapse prevention after detox is paramount, so it's important to consult your provider through the entire process and explore medication-assisted treatment to prevent relapse after detox.

FINANCIAL CONSIDERATIONS

Unfortunately, when setting realistic expectations for recovery, there's a financial aspect to be considered, and it can be a roadblock for people. The good thing is that there are many helpful programs for people who need financial assistance. My advice is to start exploring and asking questions. Medicaid is an excellent option, as it can cover medical visits and medication at no cost to the patient. Additionally, ride services can be arranged to transport patients to office visits and pharmacies at no cost. Many other programs incentivize patients to attend their visits, meaning patients receive money for just going to an appointment. Also, there are programs designed to assist individuals below a specific poverty line in obtaining a free phone and monthly phone service, ensuring they stay connected and can access necessary services. The bottom line is that resources are available. There are countless programs specifically designed to assist those in need, and with a bit of digging and asking the right questions, you can find the support you need to access addiction treatment. Don't hesitate to reach out to local health departments, non-profits, and community organizations for guidance and assistance.

At Renew Health, we have a patient success coordinator who helps people explore their options. Essentially, she does the work of a social worker. Since we're a private practice and don't have funds or resources coming from a federal or state level, we collaborate with other organizations in town. One of our collaborators in particular is Alianza of New Mexico. They help community members with harm reduction, housing needs, and other necessities.[2] For their patients struggling with addiction, they are even able to offer incentives like paying them $25 if they go to their appointments. Also, they can help patients get set up on Medicaid. Since Alianza provides particular services that we are unable to provide, we work with them and refer patients to them for supplemental help. We even have an agreement between Renew Health and Alianza in which they cover the cost of a patient's visits for the first two months if someone needs financial assistance, and it's state-funded. So even if a patient doesn't have insurance or doesn't have the ability to get insurance, they can still get two months of treatment and medication for free.

Essentially, there are systems put in place to help ensure that anyone who needs treatment can get treatment. Even if someone is struggling with addiction, and they don't live anywhere near an addiction clinic, there's a solution out there for them. It may take some research, but there's a tool on the recovery tool belt for every issue that can arise.

BALANCING IN-PERSON AND REMOTE SUPPORT

In this day and age, telehealth is an integral part of our medical system, and Renew Health is not the exception to this rule. We're able to help anyone living in all four corners of the state of New Mexico. Although I prefer seeing a patient in person, being able to shake their hand, and making that human connection, I completely understand that in-person meetings are not a feasible option for everyone. Some people live hours away or are unable to take the time off of work to drive to their appointments.

The important thing is that, whether it's telehealth or in-person, I'm able to do the exact same treatment. And most people whom I've helped through telehealth are very on the ball. They're able to learn the technology, and we're able to get their medication to their local pharmacy or shipped to their house. Even if the patient needs an injection, they're able to schedule a medical professional at their own pharmacy to do the injection. Telehealth is also a great option for in-person patients who want to supplement their regular appointments with extra online meetings or in-person patients who want to transition to telehealth once their need for frequent meetings lessens.

With anything, there are drawbacks. Telehealth sometimes makes it harder for people to hold themselves accountable for attending meetings. Also, those extra minutes in person when someone's first coming into the room or leaving for the day are invaluable when I'm trying to get to know my patients and let them know I'm in their corner. When someone's considering telehealth, it's important they understand that being on time to appointments is just as important as when they were in person, and regular meetings are still mandatory when someone is going through medication-assisted treatments.

Just recently, I was reminded of the beauty of telehealth. I got a call from Shiprock, New Mexico, which is in the far northwest corner of the state and about six hours away from Renew Health in Roswell. Apparently, this patient's mother saw one of our ads on television and gave our number to her son who was struggling with addiction. Now I have a patient in Shiprock. It makes me so excited to think of the help we can offer the state as a whole. Maybe this patient will go through with recovery, tell his buddy about us, and then that person will tell his buddy. Soon enough, we'll be able to help everyone in San Juan County just through word of mouth and telehealth. Overall, I've had great success with telehealth whether the person was addicted to alcohol, opioids, or stimulants. If they're somewhere in the state, I know I can help them out. The dream is that, someday, we can expand our services nationwide. Until then, if you're interested in telehealth, local research is the best way to start, and soon enough, you'll be on the road to recovery from the comfort of your own home.

People come into our practice with a lot of expectations: what recovery will feel like, how detox will drain them, how long they want to be on medication, and how many setbacks they will face. As a medical professional, setting expectations is essential in order to help people feel confident in their recovery. I would love every patient to know that there is one expectation that is incredibly realistic: Once you start down the road to recovery, there will be a snowball effect. Once you add positivity into your life, that positivity will multiply at astounding rates. More positivity builds motivation, which leads to more positive thoughts, which leads to better actions and more positive outcomes.

I've seen it time and time again. A patient comes into the office one week into treatment and can't believe the incredible progress they've made. They come in and say, "You wouldn't believe it."

To which I always respond, "Yes, I would believe it. That's what happens here."

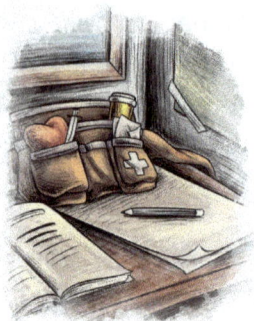

RECOVERY
WORKBENCH

Journal Prompts:

[?] What are your goals for recovery?

- What has your addiction kept you from doing? How will you use your sobriety to accomplish this goal?

- How can you measure your success beyond days of sobriety?

- Are your goals strong enough to guide you on the recovery highway?

[?] What have your experiences with detox been like?

- How do you feel about detox now?

- If you had a friend about to go through detox, what advice would you give them?

[?] When have you faced a setback in your recovery journey?

- What triggered the setback?

- How did you feel?

- What made you get back on the recovery highway?

[?] How are you going to pay for treatment?

- Are there any resources in town that can help?

[?] Fill out your goals for the corresponding time periods. What would you like to accomplish within these time frames?

	Goals
Today	
A Week	
A Month	
A Year	

TOOLS

- [✓] Medication-assisted treatment (MAT) is the treatment of substance use disorders using medications, along with counseling and therapy.

- [✓] Methadone has been a commonly used medication for opioid use disorder, but advancements in technology have made buprenorphine and naltrexone the optimal choices for recovery from opioid addiction by reducing cravings and withdrawal symptoms as well as preventing future opioid effects.

- [✓] Benzodiazepines are used for detox from alcohol use disorder, which can be incredibly dangerous and should be handled by a medical professional. Naltrexone is ideal for treating alcohol cravings and effects, but disulfiram and acamprosate are alternatives.

- [✓] While there are currently no FDA-approved medications for stimulant use disorder, off-label prescribing of naltrexone and bupropion is recommended.

- [✓] Detoxification and withdrawal remain obstacles for many trying to get sober, but medically managed withdrawal removes the barrier of pain and discomfort.

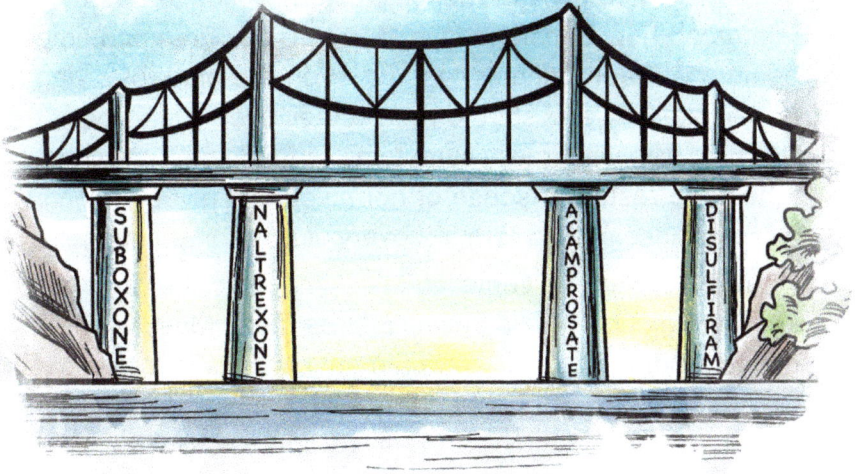

CHAPTER 4
MEDICATION-ASSISTED TREATMENT

My first exposure to medication-assisted treatment (MAT) was while I was in school to become a nurse practitioner. Seeing firsthand how unique medications could stabilize patients with specific needs and make such a significant impact on their recovery was eye-opening. It was like watching sparks of hope come alive for people who had been struggling for so long in the dark. And once that hope came alive, I watched patients thrive.

Since then, my experience at Renew Health has only reinforced how transformative MAT can be. Time and time again, I've seen patients who were on the brink of giving up find stability and start to rebuild their lives. MAT doesn't just help with withdrawal symptoms or fending off cravings; it helps to restore a sense of normalcy and gives patients a real chance at long-term recovery. It is a game-changer.

Many patients come to me with little to no prior knowledge of medication-assisted treatment. Most people's understanding of addiction treatment consists of traditional rehab or counseling, but they aren't aware that FDA-approved medications can help to address the physical aspects of addiction. On first hearing this, patients are often curious and sometimes skeptical. People believe that they are trading one substance for another. This is far from the truth. In actuality, patients are considered sober when the only drugs they are taking are prescribed for MAT.

I walk patients through the benefits and how they can make the recovery process more manageable. I explain that these medications can help reduce the cravings for a substance and minimize any symptoms from withdrawal. Patients have an easier time focusing on their recovery and goals without these stressors. I think back to the patient I met while in NP school who was excited that he was able to continue his education because of MAT. The medication was able to mitigate symptoms and keep him focused on his recovery. MAT is the cornerstone of our approach to addiction treatment, but it is not the singular solution. It's combined with counseling and behavioral therapies, embodying a holistic approach toward recovery.

MAT opens up a new possibility for patients that they often never knew existed. These medications are prescribed by medical providers and clinics around the nation. Just like someone might take insulin to help manage their diabetes, these medications help manage addiction by stabilizing brain chemistry. By educating patients about the different medications used, we can start building a treatment plan that they feel confident about and committed to. MAT isn't a one-size-fits-all solution; everyone's body reacts to medication differently. I work together with patients to find the right medication and dosage that works best for them, and we combine it with counseling and behavioral therapies to address the underlying issues of addiction.

Knowledge is potential power, and with the right information about MAT, anyone struggling with addiction can take action and continue on their journey down the recovery highway.

OPIOID USE DISORDER

Methadone

Methadone remains the most well-known medication used in medication-assisted treatment for opioid addiction, also referred to as medications for opioid use disorder (MOUD). It's a long-acting opioid agonist, which means it works by activating the same receptors in the brain that other opioids affect, but in a much more controlled and stable way. By filling the space in those opioid receptors, methadone alleviates withdrawal symptoms and reduces cravings without producing the high associated with other opioids (if taken appropriately) for about 24 hours.[1] Patients are left feeling more stable and focused, making engaging in their everyday lives and recovery plans easier.

However, there are some significant drawbacks to methadone. Methadone has the potential risk for abuse and overdose. As a full agonist, it can be addictive and dangerous if not properly managed. In some cases, individuals misuse methadone by combining it with other opioids to enhance their high, which increases the risk of overdose. Using a benzodiazepine, such as Xanax, has a similar suppressive effect on the body to methadone. If combined, the risk of overdosing and losing the drive to breathe increases. The heart rate and respiratory rate slow down until breathing stops altogether. Due to the highly controlled nature of methadone treatment, patients often have to visit a licensed opioid treatment program every single day to receive their dose, which makes it difficult to maintain a job, take care of their family, or manage other responsibilities. Returning to a clinic every day for methadone can sometimes make it feel like you're not moving forward.

Because of these issues, I tend to prefer prescribing buprenorphine (Suboxone) or naltrexone. These have a lower risk of abuse and overdose and can be prescribed on a more flexible schedule. In fact, naltrexone has *no* risk of abuse or overdose. Even though it has its limitations, methadone can be effective for some patients, especially those who have not had success with other treatments. When 87 percent of people with opioid use disorder do not receive evidence-based treatment, getting any treatment can make a huge impact on someone with OUD.[2] By preventing withdrawal and cravings, synthetic opioid compounds like methadone and buprenorphine can reduce overdoses by up to 76 percent.[3] With the right medication and comprehensive support, it could save someone's life.

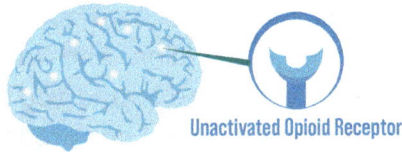

Unactivated Opioid Receptor

Methadone | Buprenorphine | Naltrexone

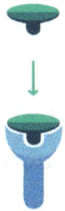

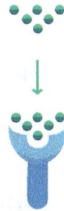

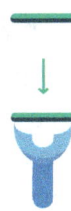

A full agonist produces a maximum effect. | *A partial agonist produces a partial effect.* | *An antagonist blocks agonists from binding.*

Medications for opioid use disorder activate receptors in the brain to achieve different effects depending on the type of treatment a patient is receiving.

My Experience with Methadone

Testimonial from a Patient at Renew Health

I was a heroin addict when I was younger. Then I got heavily into pills. Eventually, my friend told me about the methadone clinic, so I started going there. It was a lifesaver. I'm telling you, it was a *true* lifesaver.

For my treatment, they offered me Suboxone or methadone. I had no idea what Suboxone was, so I chose methadone. I was on it for six years. With methadone, there are a few drawbacks. One is that at the methadone clinic, you are treated like a child. You have to go in *every day* to get your medication.

Also, the people there don't care about you. You go in there, get your medication, and have to get the hell out. Even if you come in and you're high, they don't care. Because of that, I don't really see it as a treatment center. That being said, I was there for six years, and it did save my life. It got me off of pills, which was exactly what I needed it to do.

After six years, I got kicked out of the methadone clinic for not behaving myself, so I got sent over here to Renew Health. This is where I learned about Suboxone and found out that it's a combination of two medications: buprenorphine and naloxone. I'm telling you, I absolutely love it. *Love it.* I wouldn't change it for the world. It's true, methadone does have its place. It was great, and it really worked for me because I wanted it to work. But some people in the methadone clinic don't want it to work; they just want to get high. If they would let me go back there and counsel with those people, I would try to get them to come over to the Suboxone side because it's that awesome. I can actually live my life, not having to go to a clinic every single day. Instead, I see Trent twice a month and I'm good to go.

Even the transition from methadone to Suboxone was great, with very minimal withdrawal. My pain is managed, I don't have any cravings, I smile, and I feel good. Now, I'm 62 years old, and my biggest fear is getting high. With Suboxone, I don't have to worry about that. If I could go back six years, I would've started with Suboxone.

Buprenorphine

Buprenorphine is a partial opioid agonist. This means it only partially activates the opioid receptors in the brain, compared to full agonists like fentanyl or methadone. Because of its unique chemical structure as a synthetic opioid, buprenorphine reduces cravings and withdrawal symptoms without producing a significant high. As buprenorphine saturates the receptors, it creates a ceiling effect—meaning beyond a certain dose, taking more won't increase the effects. This built-in safety feature significantly reduces the risk of abuse and overdose. It's a much safer option for many patients compared to other opioids.

Certified providers can prescribe buprenorphine, allowing patients to take it at home instead of having to visit a clinic every day. This flexibility makes it much more convenient and less disruptive to a patient's life. By spending less time at a clinic, a patient is free to maintain a job, manage their responsibilities, and live their life. Buprenorphine is often administered as a sublingual tablet or film that dissolves under the tongue. In addition to the dissolvable tablets, a patient can receive extended-release injections, available as the prescriptions Sublocade or Brixadi. These injections are given weekly or monthly, providing a consistent dose of medication over time. This is a great option for patients who struggle with daily adherence or prefer not to take medication every day. It also reduces the risk of diversion and misuse, as the injections have to be administered by a healthcare professional.

Naltrexone

Naltrexone is another important medication used in MAT for both opioid and alcohol addiction. Like naloxone, naltrexone is an opioid antagonist. It works by blocking the opioid receptors in the brain, preventing any opioids from having an effect. If anyone tries to use opioids while on naltrexone, they won't feel the usual high they are used to.

Unlike methadone and buprenorphine, any healthcare provider can prescribe naltrexone. Patients will take naltrexone in either two forms: a daily oral tablet or a monthly injectable. The injectable form, Vivitrol, is often preferred because it ensures that the patient consistently receives the medication, eliminating the need for daily adherence. By relying on an injection once a month, it's the easiest way for a patient to be compliant with treatment. I often tell my patients, "Instead of having to make 30 decisions a month to take the pill, you can just make one decision and get the injection."

One of the benefits of naltrexone is its non-addictive qualities. The medication is not an opioid and does not have the potential for abuse. This makes it a very safe option for many patients. However, patients must be fully detoxed from opioids before starting naltrexone, as taking it too soon can cause precipitated withdrawal. Withdrawal symptoms will come on quickly from the naltrexone, disrupting the other opioids already in the opioid receptors. When administered properly, withdrawal can be easily managed.

Suboxone

The brand name drug, Suboxone, is a combination of medications: buprenorphine and naloxone. The buprenorphine does the heavy lifting, reducing cravings and withdrawal symptoms. It also has a blocking effect, keeping other opioids from binding to the receptors, reducing the effects if someone tries to use other opioids while on buprenorphine. Naloxone, on the other hand, is an opioid receptor antagonist and is included to deter misuse. Most people know naloxone as the active ingredient in Narcan, which is administered after an opioid overdose. If Suboxone is taken as prescribed, the naloxone component remains inactive. However, if someone tries to dissolve and inject the medication to get high, naloxone will kick in and fully block the opioid receptors, causing immediate withdrawal symptoms. This built-in safeguard helps reduce the potential for abuse.

Suboxone supports many people struggling with opioid addiction. It offers a balance of effectiveness, safety, and convenience, making it a preferred option in many treatment plans.

Suboxone Saved My Life
Testimonial from a Patient at Renew Health

Twenty years ago, I had a life-altering work injury. I worked for Airborne Express, and one day, while working on a smaller aircraft, I bent down to pick up a box at my feet. Picking up the box, I didn't realize how close I was to the wing locker. I backed into the wing locker really hard, and it broke my back. After that, the chronic pain pushed me onto a path of addiction to painkillers.

For my medication, I started out on hydrocodone, but the majority of my addiction career was spent taking oxycodone (15 milligrams). What I found out while taking opioids for two decades is that the more you're on it, the more you want it, and there is no quality of life. All I would do all day, every day, was sit in bed, take my medication, and then just lay there waiting until I could take it again. My doctor told me I could take the medication every four to six hours. I needed a dose every four hours to manage my pain, but I had to wait six hours because I was always in danger of running out. On good days, I would have enough energy to watch TV or do a puzzle book. But there weren't many good days.

After years of living like that, and even losing all of my teeth because of the substance abuse, I said to myself, "I'm 54 years old, and I'm tired of this." I knew I wanted to get off of oxycodone, but being an addict meant that no matter how much I *wanted* to stop taking it, I still felt like I needed my pain medication. Seeking treatment scared me. I didn't know how to do it or where to even start. That's when a close friend told me about Renew Health and her experience with Suboxone. At first, I didn't really believe her, and I was weary of medication-assisted treatment. In the past, I had tried methadone but had a bad experience with it: The withdrawal was terrible and occurred often. The doctors kept telling me that withdrawing from oxycodone wasn't going to kill me. Those words didn't alleviate the pain.

Even though I still wasn't 100 percent sure, I called Renew Health and made an appointment with Trent. The very day of my appointment, Trent told me, "If you take Suboxone today, you will feel better tonight." I took Suboxone, went to bed, and I woke up feeling good. The next morning, I woke up feeling wonderful. Now, I finally feel like myself again: I don't feel sick or have any withdrawals, and I have so much more energy than before. The most astonishing thing is that I have not craved opiates since I started Suboxone. If my back starts to hurt, I can just take a Tylenol or an Advil, and it completely takes away the pain in a way that only oxycodone did before. I can actually be productive and clean my house because I'm not tied to my bed anymore. It sounds like a small win, but a clean house is something I used to take for granted.

Renew Health is such a comforting, soothing place for me now, and everyone already knows my name. Even when I once told Trent that I slipped up, he never made me feel ashamed or embarrassed. I cried in front of him, thinking I'd let him down. I never want to let anybody down, but I felt so supported by Renew Health that I left the appointment knowing I would be strong and stay on the path of recovery. In the past, I've had doctors refuse to keep seeing me because I missed a couple of appointments. I know Trent would never do that.

Now, every time I go into the pharmacy for Suboxone, I tell them, "If you have someone whose doctor is weaning them off pain medication, please send them to Trent." I know I'll always be an addict. I also know that Suboxone has saved my life. I feel a hundred times better now than when I was on painkillers. My journey to recovery has been brief so far, but what I've gained in this short time is life-changing. I couldn't have done it without a place like Renew Health.

ALCOHOL USE DISORDER

Benzodiazepines

Alcohol detox can be especially dangerous if not handled properly. It should be monitored under the appropriate medical supervision to protect from any symptoms of alcohol withdrawal syndrome. Trying to quit cold turkey could result in death, so any patient trying to detox from alcohol should consult with a medical professional first. Don't try to push through it.

Benzodiazepines are used to combat alcohol withdrawal symptoms. For the first 6 to 12 hours, patients can expect minor withdrawal symptoms, including insomnia, anxiety, and nausea. After 12 to 24 hours, alcoholic hallucinosis might occur with visual and auditory hallucinations. Within 24 to 48 hours, patients may encounter withdrawal seizures. And after 48 to 72 hours, delirium tremens may set in, including hallucinations, disorientation, and more seizures. Benzodiazepines have been found to be most effective in treating alcohol withdrawal symptoms during these time windows as they affect gamma-aminobutyric acid (GABA) receptors similar to alcohol.[4] Their ability to reduce anxiety and help patients sleep through a large portion of their withdrawal makes them incredibly effective.

Ativan is most often used for inpatient detox to reduce symptoms and reduce discomfort. Most commonly known for its brand name, Valium, diazepam can calm patients as they go through some of the worst symptoms during outpatient treatment. It's able to suppress symptoms, reduce the risk of withdrawal seizures, and shorten the course of withdrawal.[5] Librium, or chlordiazepoxide, may also be used for outpatient care.

Naltrexone

In addition to being used to treat opioid addiction, naltrexone also reduces cravings and blocks the pleasurable effects of alcohol—it reduces the enjoyable "buzz." It does this by altering the dopamine release following alcohol use, blocking those receptors in the brain.[6] The effect helps patients maintain sobriety and resist the urge to drink.

Just like for opioid use disorder, patients can take naltrexone as a daily tablet or a monthly, extended-release injection, Vivitrol. But patients cannot be on opioids, whether prescribed or otherwise, while taking naltrexone, as it works as an opioid antagonist. For example, if a patient was taking a prescription opioid for pain after a tooth extraction, then the opioid's pain relief would be blocked by naltrexone. Also, unlike Suboxone or buprenorphine, which can trigger early withdrawal-type symptoms if stopped abruptly, naltrexone and Vivitrol do not give a physical reminder for the patient to take their medication, so it is crucial that patients adhere strictly to their prescribed medication regimen, regardless of how they physically feel.

Acamprosate

Acamprosate is used to prevent future cravings to drink. It is usually prescribed after drinking cessation and detox, but it can be taken during a medically supervised withdrawal. How acamprosate works is not totally understood, but it is believed to interact with the glutamate neurotransmitter. This reduces any prolonged withdrawal symptoms.[7]

Acamprosate is usually taken as two pills, three times a day. This is a huge barrier because it's easy to forget a dose throughout the day. For most patients, I would recommend the naltrexone extended-release injection, Vivitrol, over having to remember to take six pills every day, but if naltrexone isn't as effective for a patient, then starting acamprosate could be a better alternative. Also, for some patients, having a medication to take multiple times a day may create a positive routine and serve as a psychological reminder of one's sobriety.

Disulfiram

If neither naltrexone nor acamprosate is viable for a patient, disulfiram is an alternative for discouraging drinking—it creates an unpleasant, hangover-like feeling immediately after consuming alcohol. Disulfiram blocks the breakdown of alcohol and raises acetaldehyde levels, which cause hangovers. It does not curb alcohol cravings but rather uses this negative hangover feeling to dissuade alcohol usage.[8]

STIMULANT USE DISORDER

Medication Options

There are currently no FDA-approved medications for stimulant use disorder. Methadone, buprenorphine, and naltrexone are the only three FDA-approved medications for opioid use disorder, while naltrexone, acamprosate, and disulfiram are the only three FDA-approved medications for alcohol use disorder. However, off-label alternatives do exist for those suffering from stimulant use disorder.

Off-label prescribing is common practice, as some prescriptions have other purposes beyond their FDA approval. For stimulant use disorder, the combination of naltrexone and bupropion, an antidepressant, has been found to help reduce methamphetamine use. It's believed that naltrexone reduces the euphoric effects of the stimulant, and the bupropion targets the dysphoria—the discomfort during withdrawal.[9]

While all of these medications can be highly effective, it's important to understand their strengths—and weaknesses. These medications have potential side effects, the most common being constipation, lethargy, and nausea. It's also important to follow instructions when taking any medication. Mixing them with alcohol or other drugs could result in harmful effects. Taking Suboxone with alcohol or benzodiazepines could suppress your respiratory rate and stop your breathing. Medicine is a powerful tool, but it has to be respected and handled properly.

When treated with care, medications can make the hardest parts of recovery much more manageable. First and foremost, the physical symptoms of addiction need to be overcome—the first hurdle being detox.

DETOX

Medically managed withdrawal plays an important role during outpatient detoxification (detox). Detox is the process of removing toxic substances from the body. The body will rid itself of drugs, alcohol, and any other addictive substances—but it takes time and effort. That effort manifests in withdrawal symptoms: anxiety or depression, fatigue, nausea or vomiting, sweating or fever, mood swings, and sleep disturbances. Those symptoms can be mitigated with the help of medication.

The goal of using medication in treatment is to remove the barrier of pain and discomfort. I want my patients to feel comfortable. When someone is uncomfortable due to the detox process and feels the pain of withdrawal, they're more likely to return to using again. Being in pain does not have to be a part of the process. Though there will be discomfort, avoiding pain is possible.

When you're on opioids, and you're physically dependent because you've been doing them for a long time, you're going to go through withdrawal. It's an inevitability. But, with medication, those withdrawal symptoms can be experienced differently. When detoxing from opioids, I typically present my patients with two options:

Option A is the quickest, but the most uncomfortable. Patients will stop taking opioids immediately and begin to feel the symptoms of withdrawal. I'll have them self-assess on the clinical opiate withdrawal scale (COWS) to determine when they need to take buprenorphine.[10] This isn't necessary for stimulant and alcohol usage, but specifically for opioids and opiates. Once patients are experiencing severe enough withdrawal symptoms, they can take the medicine, and within 15 minutes, they'll start feeling better. If they take it too soon when there are still high levels of opioids in their system, they'll go into precipitated withdrawal and immediately become violently ill. The buprenorphine forces the opioids out of the receptors in the most uncomfortable way possible. In the case of naltrexone, patients need to be completely detoxed from opioids before taking the medication. I tell my patients that if they follow all the directions and take their prescriptions for MAT at the right times, detox will only feel as bad as the flu. If they go into precipitated withdrawal, they'll become painfully ill immediately.

At this point, patients will either microdose the buprenorphine or Suboxone and take small doses incrementally, allowing the medication to build up in their system.[11] Or they will macrodose and take a massive dose of medication up front. Macrodosing is typically done for patients with high opioid tolerance.[12] I prefer a hybrid approach for patients—Option B.

Option B, a micro/macro hybrid technique, allows patients to avoid severe withdrawal symptoms entirely. This has become my preferred method for treatment. We set up patients to go through detox over 7 to 10 days. I have patients take microdoses of Suboxone while they are still using opioids to introduce the medication into their system. With such small amounts, they don't go into precipitated withdrawal. After a week, they stop opioid usage entirely and take a macrodose of Suboxone immediately. With the Suboxone already in their system, there is no immediate withdrawal. If they follow the directions for the medication, they can go about their normal lives, even go to work, and never reach a point of pain or great discomfort. But they have to follow instructions. A majority of my opioid use disorder patients choose Option B and are very successful.

I do have patients who come in believing they need to go through detox before meeting with me. They'll have a miserable experience going through withdrawals on their own. I always tell them that they should have come in—I could have helped them.

Detoxing from opioids might feel like death if you try to quit abruptly on your own, but it's only painful. Detoxing from alcohol, on the other hand, can be incredibly dangerous without the proper observation and medication. Before we moved to New Mexico, my wife knew someone who decided to quit alcohol cold turkey. He tried to white knuckle it and was posting on Facebook for help, uncertain of why it was so painful. Two days later, he passed away detoxing from the alcohol. Alcohol detox should not be attempted without some form of medical care.

In the case of alcohol use disorder, I can prescribe diazepam and time it out perfectly so that the patient can detox over the weekend in the comfort of their home and only take a couple of days off from work. Diazepam is able to handle most of the withdrawal symptoms, and the patient only needs to focus on drinking lots of water and resupplying their body with all the nutrients and electrolytes it needs to recover.

Detox and withdrawal symptoms may seem scary or overwhelming. I know many patients who have faced these challenges, and their experiences often became barriers to getting treatment. However, with the right medication and a clear timeline for the future, patients can maintain their sobriety for years.

TIMELINE

It's at the front of their minds: Many patients want to know how long they'll be taking their medication. When discussing the timeline for recovery and the use of medication-assisted treatment, I emphasize that everyone's recovery journey is unique. There's no one-size-fits-all approach. The length of time a patient needs to be on medication can vary greatly depending on their individual circumstances and progress. MAT is a tool to help stabilize their lives and reduce the risk of relapse. For some, it might be a short-term solution to get through the early stages of recovery. Others may need the long-term maintenance necessary to sustain their progress. The key is to regularly reassess their treatment plan and adjust as needed, prioritizing their well-being and recovery goals.

Medication can be used to assist in a dramatic shift in a patient's life, and the success and timing of that comes down to the work they put into their recovery. My very first patient, Julia, is a great testament to the power of MAT and how quickly it can help turn your life around. When she first came into my office, she was terrified.

"Every day I wake up, I feel like I'm gonna die," she said.

Julia had a dependence. She did not want to abuse OxyContin, but she had to in order to function. She was a working professional and a single mother of a 10-year-old daughter—and she was scared *every single day* that she was going to overdose and die. Julia was a patient for under a year and a half. She never once relapsed. The last OxyContin she took was the first day she came into my office.

The buprenorphine injections helped with her cravings, but after a year, we assessed all the other external factors in her life and any possible triggers for her. We agreed she was ready to slowly start spacing out her injections every four weeks, then every six weeks, then every eight weeks. Eventually, she didn't need to come in anymore.

I'm glad I haven't seen Julia in years, but she calls to say hi from time to time and to let me know she's doing well. If for some reason she ever lapsed, she knows there are tools to help her with her recovery. On the winding highway of recovery, some patients need more time on medication. And that's okay.

The timeline of recovery can also be affected by other health conditions. In the instance of pregnant women who have an opioid use disorder and are actively using opioids, they need to be on medications. MOUDs should be taken before, during, and after the pregnancy. It's safer for the mother to undergo MAT to avoid overdosing and dying. For the baby, the opioids have the potential to harm or kill the baby. If a mother is abusing drugs, the baby could be born with withdrawal symptoms. The baby isn't born addicted, but they will have a physical dependence. Postpartum is also an important time for mothers to be on MOUDs to prevent fentanyl or other opioids from entering their breast milk. Other factors, like postpartum depression, could trigger cravings in the mother and lead to substance abuse that could harm the baby. Maintaining the treatment timeline is imperative for the safety of the mother and child.

For patients taking naltrexone or Vivitrol, I strongly encourage them to set a timeline for themselves and their prescriptions. After starting MAT, patients will experience a decrease in cravings and urges. Oftentimes, I see this lead to the belief they are ready to stop taking their medication. But this is the medication doing what it does best, and unfortunately, patients taking naltrexone may be misled by this. If they stop their medication prematurely, they will not have the right recovery tools or environment in place when those cravings return. The risk of stopping treatment too soon and relapsing is significant. Because of this, I urge patients to set a timeline (6 months, 12 months, 24 months, etc.) during which they continue to take the medication, no matter how well they feel they are doing. Starting and stopping medication always needs to be a conversation with a healthcare provider.

I view addiction as a chronic disease, similar to diabetes or heart disease. How do you treat a chronic disease? Medication. Just like if you had high blood pressure, you might need to take medication long-term to manage your condition. But you don't just take medication alone. You start to change your habits and your lifestyle; you change your diet and start exercising more. As you keep up those changes, you work with your doctor to start lowering your dose, and maybe even get off the medication entirely. It's the same with MAT for addiction. Making and maintaining those lifestyle changes can be incredibly challenging for many people. Even if you've been on Suboxone for a year and your lifestyle hasn't changed, there's nothing wrong with continuing medication if you still need it. Needing long-term medication is not a sign of failure. Instead, it's a part of managing a chronic condition.

I have a patient who is in his late 60s who has been on Suboxone for over 20 years. He's been sober that whole time, not just because of the medication's effects but because he has things in his life that are so valuable to him that he doesn't want to lose them. He has a wife, children, a house, and stability. I'm very confident if we slowly weaned him off Suboxone, he would be successful and not relapse. But he's told me on multiple occasions, "The Suboxone is insurance." He'd rather check in with me once a quarter and take his medication every day than return to where he was three decades ago. Do I believe that every patient needs this insurance for this long? No—but it's there if they think they need it.

Unfortunately, the biggest obstacle to MAT isn't necessarily the length of time on the medication but getting on the medication in the first place.

OVERCOMING BARRIERS TO MEDICATION

It's difficult enough admitting you need help with your substance use disorder, but finding the best help for you can also be a struggle sometimes. Whether the resources around you are limited, or the stigma of asking for help is too great, it may be a challenge to find medication-assisted treatment. Luckily, there are resources available if you know where to look.

Navigating the different barriers to accessing treatment depends on where you are in the country. Each state may have different rules surrounding MAT, the types of medication allowed, or where you can receive treatment. Resources from your state's health department or substance abuse agency can easily be found online, but some states have more extensive care available than others. The Substance Abuse and Mental Health Services Administration (SAMHSA), an agency within the Department of Health and Human Services (HHS), can offer guidance and support. As a national agency, their website is full of resources and information about navigating state-specific barriers to treatment.[13] The National Alliance on Mental Illness (NAMI) can also aid in finding local treatment providers.[14] These directories often include detailed information about the services offered and how to access them. Additionally, local health departments are an excellent tool for understanding what barriers you might face in your state. They are aware of local regulations, available treatment centers, and any state-funded programs that might offer you aid.

Talking directly to healthcare providers in your area is another practical step. Reach out to medical providers, clinics, or treatment centers in your state that specialize in addiction treatment. They will have firsthand experience and knowledge of the types of care offered near you and can provide advice on how to receive it. Joining a support group, either in person or online, can also connect you with the right provider or resources. Members of these groups will have their own experiences with treatment and recovery. That being said, take any negative advice you get from friends or peers with a grain of salt. Just because a person you know had a negative experience with a medication, doesn't mean you're going to have the same experience. Everybody will react to treatment differently, so talking to a medical professional about your concerns is the most imperative step.

The care you receive may not even come from a physical location around you. With the rise of telehealth, accessing treatment remotely is an option. Look into providers in your state who offer telehealth services, which will allow you to receive prescriptions and participate in counseling sessions from the comfort of your home.

If you require financial assistance, many states offer programs to aid those seeking treatment. Look into programs like Medicaid, state-funded rehab centers, or nonprofit organizations that provide grants or sliding-scale fees. Sometimes it might be necessary to seek legal advice if you're encountering further barriers to treatment. Legal aid organizations can help you understand your rights and explore any legal avenues you may pursue to get the treatment you need.

It's important to be active in your own recovery. Don't be afraid to ask for help in taking action. By seeking out resources and information, you can open up new opportunities and support that will help you. The more engaged you are, the better equipped you'll be to navigate any barriers you encounter.

🩹 🩹 🩹

I make it clear to my patients that while medication is a powerful tool, it's not a magic solution on its own. Medication can help manage cravings and withdrawal, allowing patients to focus on other aspects of their recovery, but it's only one part of a comprehensive treatment plan. Patients must participate in their recovery. Addiction is a complex condition that reaches into all areas of life, including mental health, behavior, and environment. Addressing how far it reaches requires more than just medication.

Recovery is a holistic process. Medication helps stabilize a patient's condition, but true recovery involves healing their mind, body, and spirit. By combining medication with counseling, support groups, and positive lifestyle changes, patients have the best chance of achieving long-term sobriety and a healthier, happier life.

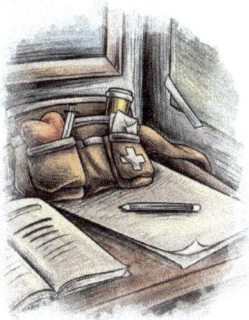

RECOVERY
WORKBENCH

Journal Prompts:

[?] Have you ever been on medication for addiction treatment before?

- If you have, how did it make you feel? Were you able to experience the benefits of the medication?

- If you haven't, how would you feel about starting a medication? Would you be nervous? How would you hope to feel?

[?] What barriers to receiving MAT have you experienced?

[?] What are some ways you think MAT can help people who are struggling with addiction?

[?] What would you tell a friend who is interested in starting MAT?

CHAPTER 5
TOOLS

☑ Many people struggling with addiction also struggle with co-occurring disorders. These need to be addressed in order to establish a holistic recovery.

☑ Whether it's cognitive behavioral therapy, family therapy, or a blend of many different types, researching and seeking talk therapy can be an essential tool on your belt.

☑ Sometimes, the road to recovery isn't just a straight path forward. Instead, uncovering strategies to reduce the harm caused by addiction can be the best way to combat addiction, allowing the tool to meet you where you're at.

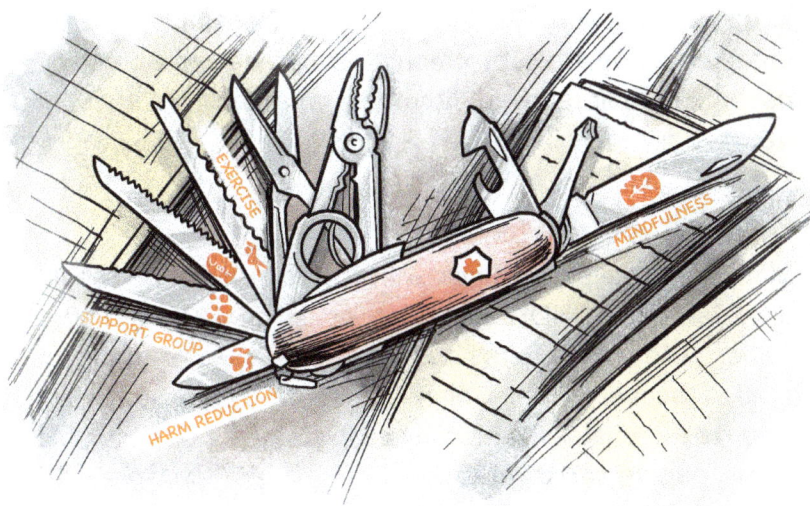

CHAPTER 5
SUPPLEMENTAL TECHNIQUES

Although medication-assisted treatment (MAT) does an abundance of work to help someone overcome addiction, science-based techniques can help someone stay on the path to recovery. At Renew Health, we believe in cognitive behavioral therapy (CBT) and counseling for every patient as well as harm reduction practices for patients who require them. It's important to make an effort to find clinics that offer more resources than just MAT to help with recovery. Addiction affects every part of a person, so it takes more than one strategy to address it. Unfortunately, mental health disorders may be a significant issue for patients who are also struggling with addiction. One doesn't necessarily cause the other, but there are supplemental resources available to aid patients in their recovery no matter what they are suffering from.

TREATING CO-OCCURRING DISORDERS

Many of my patients struggle with co-occurring mental health disorders like ADHD, depression, anxiety, PTSD, and other issues. These disorders have to be addressed when on the road to recovery, as they often feed into the addiction, which in turn exacerbates the mental health struggles. For example, some people resort to drugs when they feel depressed, and the drug use worsens the depression. This can start a severe, endless cycle. However, there are plenty of tools available to treat these disorders, including medications.

It's important that patients seek a provider or clinic that is willing to work with them in treating any co-occurring disorders. Renew Health is able to prescribe medication that will complement a patient's addiction treatment and treat any mental health disorders. While this treatment is available at Renew Health, it's important to research experts in your community who can assist you in this part of recovery. Most primary care physicians can prescribe medication for mental health, but if a patient isn't getting the right support from their doctor, they should speak with a specialist at their addiction treatment clinic or get a recommendation for either a psychiatrist or another medical expert with experience in treating mental health, like a psychiatric mental health nurse practitioner. Getting addiction treatment without treating co-occurring mental disorders is like only paddling on one side of a canoe—you'll just end up going in circles.

Once a patient receives treatment for co-occurring disorders, it's important they disclose every medication they are taking with each healthcare professional they are working with to prevent any redundancies in prescriptions. I never want to step on the toes of another healthcare provider and overprescribe a medication a patient is already receiving. However, if symptoms are still persistent over time, patients should be able to talk with their provider about upping, changing, or adding a prescription. Finding the right medication and dosages takes patience and observation.

Medication is not the only treatment for mental health disorders though. MAT and psychiatric medications working alongside CBT can break the cycle of co-occurring disorders because they help patients deal with both sides of the equation. The medications prescribed to address these disorders can be incredibly effective, but even then, therapy is encouraged alongside medication. For someone who has never talked to a healthcare professional about their mental health before, this might seem like too much all at once. It can be a daunting task to address one's mental health, whether it be depression, anxiety, or bipolar disorder, but it is necessary for a successful recovery. The stigma around mental health can be a barrier to treatment, just as addiction's stigma can prevent treatment. It takes courage to address one's behavior and make an active change, but there are therapists and specialists available all over the country.

COGNITIVE BEHAVIORAL THERAPY (CBT)

I encourage all Renew Health patients to attend at least one consultation appointment with a cognitive behavioral therapist. We have an in-house therapist at our office, but we also collaborate with other therapists in town in order to give our patients several options. The reason that CBT is so important is that, more often than not, having an addiction means having co-occurring disorders, but even patients who do not have a co-occurring disorder will benefit from adding CBT to their recovery tool belt. This is because CBT addresses ways of thinking and behavioral patterns that contribute to psychological problems. The American

Psychological Association defines the core principles of cognitive behavior therapy as follows:

1. Psychological problems are based, in part, on faulty or unhelpful ways of thinking;

2. Psychological problems are based, in part, on learned patterns of unhelpful behavior; and

3. People suffering from psychological problems can learn better ways of coping with them, thereby relieving their symptoms and becoming more effective in their lives.[1]

Because of the emphasis on thought and behavioral patterns, CBT addresses the "here and now" rather than digging into someone's past and childhood experiences. Addressing the present is paramount when recovering from addiction because it helps patients learn how to handle situations they're put in. Knowing oneself is one side of it, but that knowledge doesn't help anyone if they don't learn how to change habitual behaviors. It goes back to the concept of "knowledge is potential power." CBT helps to harness that knowledge and break the chain of addiction to start re-linking new behaviors. The medication-assisted treatment helps your body to recover from addiction, and then the CBT will simultaneously help to build new behaviors as the craving for the substance ebbs. The combination of medication and therapy allows patients to make better choices in the here and now.

I realized the importance of combining CBT with MAT early on in my career as a nurse practitioner. During my clinical rotations and subsequent practice, it became clear that while MAT was incredibly effective in managing the physical symptoms of addiction, it wasn't addressing the underlying psychological and behavioral aspects that contribute to substance use. I saw firsthand that patients who only relied on medication often struggled with the same triggers and thought patterns that led them to use substances in the first place. They needed more than just a way to manage their cravings and withdrawal symptoms; they needed tools to change their behaviors and thought processes while addressing their stressors and triggers. Some medical professionals only think, "There's a drug problem. I'm going to address the drug problem." But it's important to find help from professionals who understand that if they're not addressing the mental health side of addiction, they're not truly taking care of their patients.

It's essential to keep in mind that, for some patients, depression and anxiety might not be pre-existing conditions but rather symptoms of the transition into recovery. When patients are going through detox and first starting on the road to recovery, these feelings of depression and anxiety can feel heightened as their body adjusts. Typically, those symptoms will spike at first, but then they will plateau and eventually start to go down.

Although every patient can gain insight from cognitive behavioral therapy, there are certain things patients say that communicate to me that CBT will be especially beneficial for them. For instance, if a patient frequently mentions feeling overwhelmed by stress or unable to cope with their emotions, that's a strong indicator. Statements like "I don't know how to handle my anxiety without using" or "I always end up in the same situations" are signals that CBT could be very helpful. Another indicator is when patients talk about persistent negative thought patterns or self-beliefs, such as "I'm not worth saving" or "I'll never be able to stay clean." These kinds of thoughts can be deeply ingrained and contribute to ongoing substance use. I also pay attention to patients who struggle with impulsive behaviors or who feel trapped in a cycle of using and relapsing. They might say things like "I don't think before I act" or "I can't kick the habit." Basically, whenever a patient expresses feelings of being stuck, overwhelmed, or trapped by their thoughts and behaviors, it's a strong sign that CBT could offer significant benefits. It's about giving them the tools to understand and change the patterns that contribute to their addiction, leading to a more sustainable recovery.

For patients who have experienced detox and recovery many times before, I highly recommend CBT because even though they are well-versed in the process, it's clear to me they're in a cycle and need extra support to make their recovery last long term. I had a patient who walked me through exactly how her body would react to the detox process. She even knew the exact hour that detox would be at its worst. I would argue that patients like her *need* the support of cognitive behavioral therapy for long-lasting, positive change. No matter a patient's experience level with recovery, I always talk to them about CBT and tell them to do their own research.

To encourage them, I use the same technique when trying to get someone to try medication-assisted treatment for the first time. I say to them, "Just give it a shot. Worst-case scenario: You hate it, and you go right back to what you're doing right now. Or best-case scenario: You love it, and you pick up some new tips, tricks, and ways to approach your journey."

I also emphasize that just one meeting with a therapist can be a game-changer for their recovery. An appointment with a mental health specialist can introduce patients to the methods utilized in CBT and other approaches to therapy. These are tools to add to the recovery tool belt. As they progress through treatment, patients understand how their thoughts, emotions, and behaviors are all connected. A single meeting with a therapist has the potential to open a patient's eyes to how thought patterns contribute to their addiction—and how they have the power to change those patterns. A kind and caring therapist is able to build trust with a patient and encourage them to continue with therapy. A non-judgmental environment and an introduction to simple CBT tools can kickstart healthier coping strategies and reframe thoughts. Even simple techniques learned in an initial meeting can make a big difference in how they manage stress, cravings, and negative emotions.

Despite the benefits, I am also very cognizant of hesitations that people may have when considering CBT or any type of therapy. One of the primary barriers is the stigma associated with mental health treatment. Patients worry about what others will think, or they misunderstand who can benefit from CBT. Some people think that therapy is only for people with severe mental problems, rather than something anyone can come away from with a positive experience and a new lease on life. The list of barriers can feel endless: money considerations, time constraints, lack of available therapists, a fear of opening up, etc. To many, it can feel like an uphill battle not worth taking on.

For those who are unsure due to any number of these reasons, my first piece of advice is to keep an open mind. It's natural to feel uncertain about trying something new, especially when it comes to therapy. However, CBT has helped many people make significant improvements in their lives, and it's worth exploring how it might benefit you. I tell people to do their own research. To start researching, I recommend beginning with reputable sources online. Websites like the American Psychological Association (APA) and the National Institute of Mental Health (NIMH) offer detailed information about what CBT is, how it works, and the types of issues it can help address. These resources provide a solid foundation of knowledge and can help dispel any myths or misconceptions. Even online forums like Reddit can help people reach out to others who have shared their own experiences online and start a conversation. Reading books and articles written by experts in the field can also be very informative. Another great way to learn about CBT is by listening to podcasts or watching videos that feature therapists and individuals who have undergone CBT. Hearing real-life stories and experiences can make the concepts more relatable and easier to understand.

Healthcare providers and therapists can offer personalized information based on your specific situation and answer any questions you might have. Remember, taking the first step to learn more about CBT can be empowering. The more you understand, the better equipped you'll be to make an informed decision about whether it's the right approach for you. Get on websites, make phone calls, ask questions, and educate yourself. There are so many mental health resources out there. Finding the right combination for you and your needs is paramount for long-lasting recovery.

Family therapy is also good for patients whose families are deeply involved in their recovery or for patients who want their families to be more involved. Addiction affects every person in the family; it's not something that only lands on the individual patient. When wanting to create a more supportive environment with constructive communication, family therapy can be indispensable. Many patients feel like their families don't understand what they're going through, and it's important to bridge those gaps. Understanding addiction is the only way forward when supporting a loved one.

Beyond CBT and family therapy, there are so many different types of therapy that can be beneficial. I also highly recommend group therapy. Group therapy provides a supportive environment where individuals can share their experiences and learn from others who are going through similar struggles. It promotes a sense of community and reduces feelings of isolation, which can be very powerful in the recovery process. Other types of therapy include contingency management (CM), dialectical behavior therapy (DBT), trauma-informed therapy, mindfulness-based therapy, and family systems therapy.

No matter which type of therapy is right for you, if you're struggling with an addiction, it can be extremely helpful to not only talk to your provider about medication-assisted treatment but also to a therapist about the certain thought patterns and behaviors that hinder your recovery. Ask for help, and allow the process to be as easy as possible for yourself.

Treatment Toward a Durable Recovery

Dr. Bob Phillips, Emeritus Coordinator of Human Services and Addiction Studies, Eastern New Mexico University–Roswell

The establishment of Renew Health by Trent Carter was a gratifying and timely addition to the fairly limited array of addiction treatment services in our area. Renew Health is our community's first full-service healthcare provider of medication-assisted treatment services. In addition to providing treatment in my own practice, I make active referrals and arrange continuing care, including MAT for patients. There is robust evidence for the use of specialized medications in effectively treating substance use problems, most effectively in combination with behavioral and social interventions.

In the United States, the median length of an "addiction career" (the timespan from first usage to the first year of recovery) is 27 years.[2] A primary barrier to treatment remains the negative stigma surrounding substance use problems and addictions. Nonetheless, substance use disorders are strikingly similar to other chronic health conditions, including diabetes, hypertension, asthma, and heart disease, both in terms of their treatability and potential for recovery. There are nearly 23 million persons in the US currently in successful long-term recovery.[3] Among those who have been treated for addiction, addiction careers are shortened to a median of nine years.[4]

Recovery is most effective when behavioral treatments (like therapy), social supports (including family therapy and 12-step group participation), and pharmaceutical treatments are used in combination. While research shows that pharmaceutical treatments are reasonably effective on their own, particularly with opiate dependence, outcomes are improved when treatments are combined. Although some may hesitate to participate, there is now substantial research evidence for making Alcoholics Anonymous, Narcotics Anonymous, or other 12-step/mutual aid communities an active part of one's recovery efforts.[5] An emerging number of faith-based recovery fellowships are now commonly available as well.

Addiction is rarely the only issue patients face in recovery. People present with any number of co-occurring disorders that need more than just addiction medications for treatment. These include depression, anxiety, trauma, sleep disorders, and family or marital problems. Resolving these co-occurring concerns may be essential in supporting recovery and preventing relapse. Family therapy and marital counseling can help heal relationships because addiction so often does harm to family members, friends, and peers.

In considering what types of treatment may be right for you, it's important to know that most therapists don't adhere to a single form or modality. Many providers today may work from a cognitive-behavioral framework but will blend strategies or practices from a number of different schools or models. For example, much of my work is consistent with the practices of motivational interviewing (MI) and solution-focused therapy (SFBT). Through MI, a therapist or counselor guides patients to implement change on their own terms. SFBT is a brief, evidence-based form of therapy that is goal-oriented and focused more on potential solutions rather than problems.

A more important predictor of outcome than the model of treatment utilized is the actual strength of the client/therapist working alliance or therapeutic relationship. A patient and a provider should have a good rapport. There must be trust, an agreement on goals and approaches, as well as a sense of partnership with one another. Other important predictors include one's level of hope and optimism, commitment to change, and sufficient support, opportunities, and relationships to help make recovery possible.

Before anything else, you need to become aware that a problem exists and have reasons to change. If you are seeking help at Renew Health or any other treatment center, you likely have considered this already. It can be helpful to complete a screening questionnaire to help detect these issues, either online or with a provider.[6] Many behavioral health providers are now familiar with a very helpful approach called SBIRT, or screening, brief intervention, and referral to treatment. SBIRT interviews typically take less than 30 minutes and help identify potential problems, set recovery goals, and accomplish a "warm handoff" of the patient to appropriate resources for further assessment or treatment. A good assessment can confirm (or rule out) a substance use problem, establish an accurate diagnosis, and arrange for the appropriate type of care. Providers should be willing to take an active role in making referrals, such as helping to make appointments and consulting with the referral resources. Simply providing a patient with a business card or phone number is less helpful.

Selection of treatments will vary depending on a patient's preferences, goals, and the severity of their condition. Very few people are capable of changing their lives without formal treatment. Some will benefit from self-help interventions, brief therapy, or outpatient services. Even still, there are plenty who will need medical assistance with addiction treatment medications. This includes careful withdrawal management or potential addiction residential care. Seldom are there quick fixes, but there is always the possibility of engaging in a well-networked system of care. Just as certain, there are clearly many pathways to recovery. Guilt, shame, and despair are frequent roadblocks, yet there doesn't need to be shame surrounding recovery, including the integration of behavioral health services and medical care.

Addiction is a chronic, but effectively treatable, condition—and we should hold the same attitudes towards it that we do for any other chronic health condition. Taking Suboxone to assist with opioid dependency has parallels to taking insulin for diabetes.

Unfortunately, the use of medications to assist with recovery was viewed negatively by many providers and patients for an unnecessarily long period of time. With better evidence and professional experience today, most addiction and mental health counselors are quite open to MAT, helping to destigmatize its usage. This promotes the combination of behavioral and pharmaceutical treatments to create more certain and durable recoveries for patients.

Some people will need only minimal assistance, while others will benefit from creating a long-term system of care to support recovery over a lifetime. In the US, the median number of episodes of care before durable recovery is achieved is two. In more severe conditions, it may require additional care. The message here is: Don't give up!

Whatever the case in your personal experience, your healing path to recovery can begin now, and we wish you all success on the journey ahead.

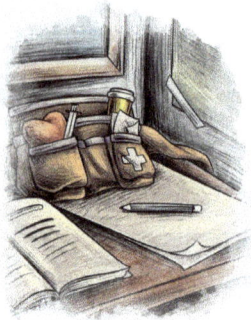

RECOVERY
WORKBENCH

Journal Prompts:

[?] Do you have a co-occurring mental disorder? If so, write about your journey and the ways in which it has affected your life.

- How could working on your co-occurring disorder help you on your path to recovery?

[?] Have you ever tried cognitive behavioral therapy before?

- If so:
  - How did it help you?
  - What made you want to start therapy?
- If not:
  - How could it help you?
  - What are the behaviors that you want to break?
  - What are the thought patterns that you want to break?

[?] Is there a type of therapy that most interests you?

[?] Do you have a stigma against therapy? If so, where does this stigma stem from?

[?] Do you know anyone in your life who has benefited from therapy or who could benefit from therapy?

HARM REDUCTION

Depending on the circumstances of a patient's visit to Renew Health, sometimes it's integral to talk to them about harm reduction practices. Many haven't heard of harm reduction before or can't conceptualize why it can be a life-saving supplemental technique. Harm reduction is a set of strategies aimed at minimizing the negative consequences of drug use, focusing on improving health and safety rather than solely eliminating drug use. The goal is to support individuals, regardless of whether the person is ready or able to stop using drugs.

Harm reduction can take on many different forms. It's important to seek harm reduction counseling in order to figure out if it's right for you. Harm reduction counseling offers non-judgmental guidance, helping individuals make informed choices about their substance use, including safer use practices and overdose prevention. The strategies include needle exchange programs, which provide clean needles or syringes to reduce the spread of infectious diseases like HIV and hepatitis C, as well as offering a safe disposal of used needles. Additionally, these programs give out clean mouthpieces and pipes and provide an opportunity for supervised injections, mitigating the risk of overdose. Naloxone (more commonly known as Narcan) distribution is another crucial strategy, as Narcan can reverse opioid overdoses. Also, harm reduction can mean providing test kits so that people can test their drugs to make sure they aren't laced with something more deadly, like fentanyl. Kits like these are often available through the health department. Your local health department is a great source as many provide information on safe drug use practices, overdose prevention, and available resources, empowering individuals to make safer choices.

Addressing housing and social services is also integral to harm reduction. Providing stable housing and access to healthcare and support services helps individuals achieve greater stability and improves their overall quality of life. Harm reduction can also mean continuing to do drugs until the patient is safely able to detox. Sometimes, if someone is waiting for their insurance to kick in or on a waitlist for inpatient detox, the best-case scenario is to have them keep doing the addictive drug. In these situations, it's important to keep follow-up appointments and keep them as accountable as possible. This minimizes the negative consequences associated with drug use, especially when immediate cessation is not possible or practical. Attempting to quit abruptly can lead to severe withdrawal symptoms or risky behavior. The goal is to keep them as safe and healthy as possible until they can access the full spectrum of treatment services. For people struggling with alcoholism, this is especially the case, as abruptly stopping the consumption of alcohol can be deadly. But if I can help someone to just have 10 beers a week instead of 60 beers a week, then that's harm reduction, and that's a win.

I don't talk to every patient about harm reduction. Rather, I bring it up as an option if I can tell they're hesitating about medication-assisted treatment or if certain harm reduction practices pertain to their life. If someone's open to MAT and consistently coming to appointments, I typically don't mention harm reduction because we can just start treatment, unless I think it might still be necessary. If they're standoffish, unsure, missing many appointments, or just seem like they don't want to be there at all, I talk them through harm reduction so that I can meet them where they are and help as much as I can with what they're willing and able to do.

Other factors help inform the harm reduction counseling I provide patients. I make sure to emphasize fentanyl test strips for people who use meth. Because fentanyl is an opioid, if someone does meth that is opioid-laced, they could overdose accidentally if their body isn't used to opioids. For that reason, talking about testing drugs to make sure they're not laced is a conversation that needs to happen. It's knowledge that everyone should have.

When it comes to harm reduction, I believe there is no more important tool than Narcan, the opioid antagonist that can treat narcotic overdose in an emergency situation. It comes in two forms: injectable and nasal spray.[7] I prescribe it to *every single one* of my patients, whether they ask for it or not. Narcan can be the difference between life and death. I made the decision early on at Renew Health to give it to each of my patients because I am deeply committed to ensuring my patients' safety and well-being and know that Narcan has the potential to save lives. Prescribing Narcan to all my patients is important to me because overdoses can happen unexpectedly, even to those who are in recovery or using lower doses. By making sure that every patient has access to Narcan, I'm giving them and their loved ones a tool that can save a life and offer essential peace of mind. If a patient says they don't want it, I tell them, "You can keep it, give it to a friend, or give it to a loved one. You can even give it to me, and I'll hand it out. It's not going to cost you anything. Please pick it up and then utilize it in some form or fashion." Especially for loved ones, I can see the peace of mind settle in when I prescribe Narcan. Now they know that if their loved one overdoses, they can do something about it.

It's also a way to empower my patients and their support networks. It empowers them with the knowledge that they can respond during an emergency. In the end, prescribing Narcan to each of my patients is essential to harm reduction and comprehensive care. This practice acknowledges the reality that overdoses happen and provides indispensable peace of mind.

WHAT TO DO IN CASE OF A SUSPECTED
OPIOID EMERGENCY

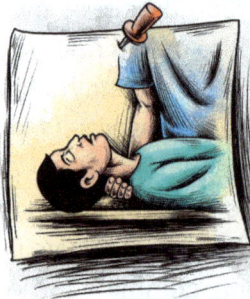

LAY

Check for slowed breathing or unresponsiveness.
Lay the person on their back and tilt the head up.

SPRAY

Insert device into either nostril and press plunger firmly.

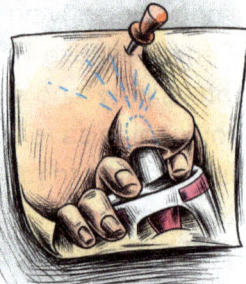

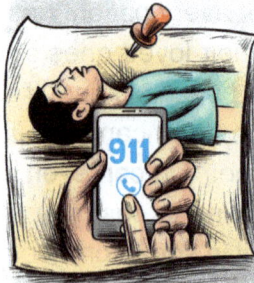

STAY

Call 911 immediately and continue to administer doses as needed.

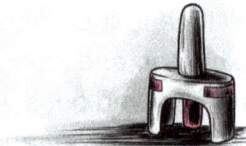

While many of my patients have benefitted from harm reduction, one story stands out in particular. Trevor struggled with heroin use, and when he first came to Renew Health, he wasn't at a point in his recovery where he was willing to explore medication-assisted treatment. We explored harm reduction strategies like needle exchange programs and Narcan to mitigate any harm associated with his drug use. Trevor's story stands out because he eventually used the Narcan I prescribed him to save his friend's life. After that, Trevor's trust in harm reduction skyrocketed, so he began attending harm reduction counseling. Through counseling, Trevor developed a better understanding of his triggers and started to implement techniques to reduce his use gradually.

After a while, Trevor attended support groups, where he connected with others who shared similar experiences. Over time, he moved from harm reduction to exploring MAT. Unfortunately, I haven't seen Trevor in a while. But his story is one of great success, even if it only lasted for a few months.

Not every story is one of success. Years ago, I had a patient who came in seeming depressed and extremely lethargic. It turned out that he had seven funerals to go to in just one week. Some of his friends had a party in which seven people overdosed on fentanyl and died. In situations like these, there are no words. But it strengthens my resolve to reach as many people as I can to tell them about harm reduction, and to distribute life-saving tools like Narcan. If everyone knew about harm reduction practices and understood how they could save lives, rather than mistrusting continued drug use as a strategy, the world would be a safer place, and people would be more likely and less ashamed to seek help.

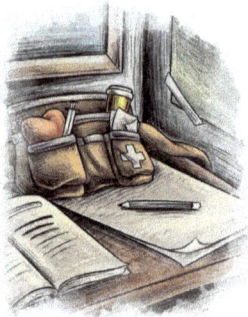

RECOVERY
WORKBENCH

Journal Prompts:

[?] Have you ever benefited from harm reduction practices?

[?] Do you know anyone whose life was saved because of harm reduction?

[?] What harm reduction programs do you think would benefit your community?

CHAPTER 6
TOOLS

- ☑ Becoming sober is a huge step in recovery, but *staying* sober can be tricky if you don't take the necessary steps to heal every aspect of your life.

- ☑ Going on walks, eating cleaner, and other ways in which you take care of your physical health will allow your body to heal from addiction and hopefully will perpetuate a new, healthy hobby.

- ☑ Having your daily and weekly goals written down will help you stay on top of your new routines and help these routines become habits.

- ☑ Recovering from addiction means you've given yourself a raise because you don't need to spend money on the substance anymore. It's important to be intentional about what you do with this extra income and to invest it in yourself and your loved ones.

- ☑ Lack of quality sleep can be a motivator for some to turn to substances, and it can also be a result of having an addiction. Getting your sleep back on track is a huge advantage when it comes to staying on the road to recovery.

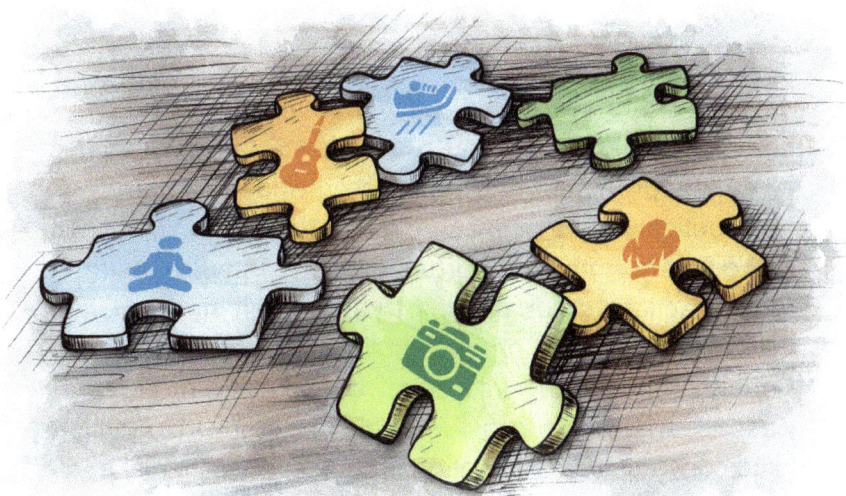

CHAPTER 6
HEALING WITH HOBBIES, HABITS, AND INTERESTS

When on the road to recovery, there are small things you can do every day in order to stay on track. Whether it's taking care of your physical health, setting small goals, managing finances, connecting with friends, or focusing on getting a good night's sleep, there are many avenues in which you can improve your life and make staying sober as easy as possible. When recovery feels hardest, strengthening these other avenues will create a recovery safety net and make life after substance abuse incredibly fulfilling.

PHYSICAL AND MENTAL HEALTH

Most patients have mixed reactions when I first introduce them to holistic life-healing practices. Some are eager to try new approaches and embrace the idea, while others are skeptical or hesitant, especially if these practices seem very different from their current lifestyle. I usually bring up these practices gradually and try to keep it simple. Often, instead of using the phrase "holistic life-healing," I'll say, "hobbies, habits, and interests," because it's more easily grasped and tailored to the specific person. During our initial conversations, I mention that recovery isn't just about stopping drug use but also about improving their overall well-being. I talk about how small changes in diet, incorporating a bit of exercise, practicing mindfulness, or diving into a hobby can significantly impact their recovery journey.

It's important to really emphasize these holistic practices once patients have stabilized on MAT and are more comfortable with the initial phases of their recovery. This is usually a few weeks into treatment. At this point in recovery, they're often more open to trying additional strategies to support their new way of life. From my experience, patients who incorporate these holistic practices along with MAT often see better outcomes. They report feeling more energetic, less stressed, and more in control of their cravings. In fact, "experts think regular physical activity can act as a healthy stand-in for addictive substances because exercise and drugs of misuse work on similar parts of your brain. They both activate your reward pathway, which triggers the release of feel-good chemicals like serotonin and dopamine."[1] Exercise and healthy eating help them build a balanced lifestyle, which reduces the chances of relapse—and to reap the benefits, it can be as simple as going on a walk.

On the flip side, patients who rely solely on MAT without engaging in holistic practices often miss out on these additional benefits. MAT helps with cravings and mitigates withdrawal symptoms, but it doesn't aid patients with stress, overall physical health, or mental issues. Holistic healing practices are imperative for the foundation of a long-term recovery. Creating a balanced lifestyle that supports both their physical and mental health will help them to thrive in their journey.

Of course, when I tell patients about healthier ways to live their lives, it's not the first time they've heard of these tactics. Our society, our news, our TV shows, and our everyday conversations are saturated with conversations about healthy living. Because of this, people know what they *should* be doing, but they often don't know *how* to do it. It's hard for some of my patients to conceptualize how to incorporate these tactics into their own lives. That's why I strive to have open and honest conversations with them to guide them through a personalized plan. A great example of this is a conversation I had with one of my patients, Will.

Will really struggles with anxiety, especially in social settings that involve big, open environments. He wanted to get back in shape, but because of his anxiety, he was terrified to go to the gym. A lot of Will's anxieties stem from his time in prison. When talking to me about it, Will said, "I know how to stay in shape. I was in shape in prison because I used to work out in my cell, but every time I think about going to the gym . . . I just can't do it."

I knew that getting Will back to work on his physical health would not only be good for his recovery, but would also be an amazing step in his mental health journey. Will knew how to get in shape, and he knew that he wanted to experience the freedom of going to the gym now that he was out of prison, but he struggled with large, open social settings. The anxiety would overwhelm him being surrounded by so many new people. He didn't know how to get over the mental roadblock of "I just can't do it." So I started talking to Will about implementing baby steps. I told him that, first, he just needs to get dressed for the gym every day. He doesn't even have to go outside; he just has to wear the same clothes he would wear at the gym. It's important to do the baby steps every day to tell the mind that you're forming a new habit. After a while, I told him to start driving to the gym. He didn't have to get out of the car or even park, but I wanted him to practice driving there, looking at it, and getting a feel for the environment. Then, I told him to eventually work his way up to parking at the gym and thinking about going inside—just reflecting. This habitual routine would eventually culminate in going inside. The first few times he goes inside, I told Will he doesn't have to work out at all. I just wanted him to walk in and familiarize himself with the building and the people.

It may sound like strange behavior, but with these baby steps, it's easier for someone to work their way up to doing something that they think is scary. The idea is that after a while, Will is going to eventually think, "You know what? I'm tired of just going into the gym and walking out. I'm actually going to work out this time." It's a very drawn-out process, but it works. It was so clear to me that Will had a willingness to go to the gym, but he just needed a little extra help getting into the right headspace. Going the extra mile as a medical provider is a huge passion of mine, so I push all of my patients to go out of their comfort zones, and they're always amazed at what they can accomplish.

For Will, getting over his fear helped his confidence and helped him grow in many other areas. Getting more comfortable with going to the gym also helped him with going to the grocery store, even though that's not what he or I set out to do. Grocery stores can also be hard for people who were incarcerated because there are people everywhere, shoppers are whipping around the aisles, and it's easy to feel like they have to be on their guard the entire time. Learning how to handle stressful situations when recovering from addiction, time in prison, or any other life-altering situation is a huge win and, sometimes, all it takes are some simple baby steps that eventually turn into a full sprint.

While stressful situations are common on the road to recovery, stress is also a common *cause* of substance addiction; people often use substances to cope with stress. These holistic life techniques give people new positive habits to cope with tense moments. Of course, the MAT will help and the CBT will help, but learning day-to-day practices sometimes means the difference between staying sober and relapsing when triggers arise.

At times, the right amount of stress can be a good thing because it can be what brings people into treatment. People who come to my practice are typically incredibly stressed due to fears of losing a job, losing a relationship, or losing their lives. This stress can drive people to want to improve their chances. But there needs to be a balance; too much stress during treatment can drive people to relapse. People often relapse because of the stress of not knowing what to do with their life after recovery, especially if they've been relying on substances for so long. When patients want to get off of MAT after they've been sober for a long time, it's important for me to make sure they have techniques put in place to mitigate stress and refill their lives in meaningful ways. Like my patient, Kenny, who came to Renew Health because he was addicted to meth. With MAT, I helped him through detox and into recovery. For that extra mile, though, Kenny got really interested in working out. Two weeks before he sought treatment, he was suicidal. Now, years later, he's absolutely shredded, off of drugs, and has aspirations to become an entrepreneur.

Another aspect that I like to focus on is maintaining a balanced and nutritious diet. Proper nutrition can drastically impact mood, energy levels, and overall mental health, which are all critical during recovery. Encouraging patients to develop healthy eating habits and perhaps even learning to cook can be therapeutic and beneficial for their physical and mental well-being. I never promote a specific diet—just eating better and eating clean. Again, this is the forging of new hobbies. If patients cook their own meals, they are learning a new skill and maybe discovering a new interest. Also, if they have kids, it's great to be able to cook for their children. Hopefully, this can help strengthen their family unit and keep them on track in recovery. Whether it's eating better or getting active, breaking down these new habits by days and weeks always makes it more attainable.

DAILY AND WEEKLY PLANNING

Daily and weekly planning strategies are essential tools for creating structure and stability in a patient's recovery journey. It provides them with a sense of routine. When someone is in recovery, having a structured plan can make a huge difference in managing their time, reducing stress, and staying focused on their goals. It helps them break down their recovery journey into manageable steps, making it less overwhelming and more achievable.

Another added benefit of a daily and weekly plan is that it ensures the activities patients engage in are helpful for their recovery, like exercising, mindfulness, and therapy, all while avoiding activities that could be potential triggers. Our patient success coordinator at Renew Health is in charge of helping patients develop daily and weekly plans and adjusting them as needed. The coordinator also assists patients in finding housing, accessing financial assistance, and connecting with support groups or community programs. This support can make a huge difference in a patient's recovery. Throughout the recovery process, the coordinator regularly checks in with patients to track their progress and address any concerns. These check-ins can be in person, over the phone, or via telehealth. Regular follow-ups help keep patients engaged and motivated. When researching different addiction centers near you, asking if they have a patient success coordinator is a good idea to ensure that the clinic goes above and beyond for each patient's holistic life-healing.

When a patient first starts treatment, every moment matters to keep them on track. Sometimes, it truly is minute-to-minute or hour-to-hour. Because of this, daily tasks are most important at the beginning of treatment, so I like to try and keep my patients as busy as possible. Here is an example of a daily schedule for a patient who is interested in holistic life-healing through habits, hobbies, and interests. In the third column, make it your own by writing about how you can incorporate these things into your own daily routine.

Daily Routine Example:

	Example	How can you incorporate this into your life?
Morning Routine:	Start the day with mindfulness practices such as meditation, journaling, or a short walk.	
Physical Activity:	Incorporate exercise, whether it's a gym session, yoga, or a simple home workout.	
Healthy Meals:	Plan and prepare nutritious meals to maintain physical health and energy levels.	
Support Meetings:	Attend any scheduled therapy sessions or support group meetings.	
Personal Development:	Dedicate time to a hobby, learning a new skill, or reading.	
Evening Routine:	Wind down with relaxing activities such as a warm bath or stretching.	
Going to Bed:	It's important to go to sleep at the same time every night, no matter if it's a weekday or a weekend.	

Weekly tasks become more important when patients are further along in their recovery and when they're ready to look at the bigger picture. Just as important as daily tasks, weekly tasks cover routines that are only required once a week. Here is an example of a weekly schedule for a patient in recovery. Once again, in the third column, make it your own by writing about how you can incorporate these things into your own weekly routine.

Weekly Routine Example:

	Example	How can you incorporate this in your life?
Review and Set Goals:	Reflect on the past week's achievements and challenges, and set goals for the upcoming week.	
Grocery Shopping and Meal Prep:	Plan and shop for healthy meals and prepare food in advance to ensure consistent nutrition.	
Social Connections:	Schedule time to connect with supportive friends or family members.	
Self-Care Activities:	Plan for self-care activities such as a nature walk or creative interests.	

Household Chores:	Include time for cleaning and organizing to maintain a healthy living environment.	
Check-In with Support Network:	Regularly communicate with a sponsor, mentor, or therapist to discuss progress and challenges.	

It's important to note that these daily and weekly tasks are always subject to change. As patients move through the recovery process, adjusting these strategies based on their evolving needs and goals is crucial. This involves regular check-ins to assess what's working and what isn't and being flexible enough to make necessary changes. For instance, if a patient finds a particular routine monotonous or unhelpful, we might introduce new activities or modify existing ones to keep them engaged and motivated. Also, as patients grow more confident in their recovery, I gradually increase the complexity and scope of their tasks, encouraging them to take on new challenges and responsibilities. This adaptive approach ensures that the planning strategies remain relevant and practical, supporting continuous growth and long-term success in their life.

For my patients, I hold them accountable for sticking to their plans, but it's done in a supportive and encouraging way. During our visits, we review their plans together and discuss any challenges they might have faced in sticking to them. It's not about punishing them but rather about helping them develop the skills and habits that will support their long-term recovery. By holding patients accountable, they learn to take responsibility for their actions and become more proactive in their recovery process. This accountability, combined with structured planning, helps them build confidence in their ability to manage their recovery and make positive changes in their lives. The goal is to empower them to take control and create a balanced, healthy lifestyle.

These conversations are paramount in the first month of treatment when I'm seeing patients weekly. When I walk into the room, I always say, "How's it going? Tell me about last week." During this stage, self-reflection between appointments is extremely important for someone struggling with addiction. If there have been setbacks, we talk about them and adjust the treatment plan accordingly. Once someone switches to monthly visits, this aspect doesn't change. It's always going to be necessary to take a moment and reflect on how things have been going and how we can promote positive momentum going forward. One of my patients, Brooke, recently found out that her mother was diagnosed with stage four terminal cancer. Brooke has been seeing me through telehealth for about a year now and has done an incredible job of sticking to her treatment. When she told me about her mom, she said, "I want to use so badly. I'm not going to. It's not the right choice to make. But I want to." I was so proud of her for being so mature in telling me how she was really feeling due to these stressful, external situations in her life that she had no control over. Even though I'm sure it was hard for her to admit her desire to relapse, I'm so glad that she did because we were able to have a conversation about it, and I could be there for her while she was reflecting on those feelings. Having honest conversations about your mindset and your ability to complete the goals you have set for yourself is essential to keep moving forward on the recovery highway.

When someone tells me that they missed a goal or task, I work with them to try to dissect what's going on and continue to motivate and encourage them to try again the next day. Some healthcare providers just want to give everyone a generic piece of advice and send them on their way, but I don't operate that way because I know that everyone's recovery story is unique. Everyone has their own past that they bring to every appointment. I think it's important for providers to go above and beyond for their patients. Finding a medical professional who is willing to go beyond prescribing medications, who is willing to take that extra five minutes with you to check in, and who is willing to offer more help than expected is invaluable and something worth searching for when looking at your options. The ability to be comfortable with talking to your provider about uncomfortable subjects can make all the difference.

FINANCIAL MANAGEMENT

During the first meeting with a patient afflicted with addiction, I always make sure to tell them the good news: "You're about to get a pay raise!" This frequently makes them laugh, but it's true; not spending money on drugs significantly reduces weekly spending. More than that, having a strong grasp of financial wellness is another area to take into consideration when talking about holistic life-healing. Being able to keep a job means getting out there, contributing to society, and having more things to hold you accountable in your sobriety. If you have a valuable job that you love, a boss that you don't want to let down, or kids who are relying on you to buy them school supplies next week, you're more likely to stay on the recovery journey so that you don't lose the financial security.

I've seen some remarkable transformations in patients' lives once they're able to focus on a job. Having a job helps patients develop a routine and gives them something positive to focus on, which are crucial elements in the recovery process. It keeps them busy and less likely to dwell on cravings or negative thoughts. Also, when patients are working, they start to regain their self-esteem and confidence. They feel proud of their contributions and the progress they're making, which boosts their overall mood and motivation.

Having financial stability and a steady income allows patients to meet their basic needs, support their families, and reduce financial stress, which can be a significant trigger for relapse. And again, framing addiction recovery as a pay raise is a powerful way to help patients see the financial benefits of sobriety. When they're no longer spending money on substances, they suddenly find themselves with more disposable income. I encourage patients to think about how they can use this extra money to improve their lives, whether it's saving for the future, investing in their education, or simply enjoying activities with friends that they couldn't afford before.

STAYING CONNECTED

Developing strong interpersonal relationships and engaging in social activities can be incredibly beneficial as a way to fill a void that substances leave in your life. Building a supportive social network through support groups, clubs, or community activities helps combat feelings of isolation and provides a sense of belonging and accountability. These relationships can offer encouragement, a space to share in successes, and support during challenging times.

I've always believed that the quickest way to change yourself is to change the people around you. If the people you normally surround yourself with are the ones selling you drugs or encouraging your continued drug use, it's imperative to surround yourself with new people who uplift you in this new chapter of your life that you're writing. When my patients push against this idea by saying, "I don't know anybody else," I just tell them to try something new. I tell them to go volunteer or go find an activity that they love. It doesn't have to cost money. I tell them to just find a way to put themselves out there. I know that it's easier said than done, but more often than not, these patients start meeting great people and building better relationships with people who are committed to helping them stay in recovery. Recovery doesn't always "take a village," but having a couple of townspeople who care about you is so valuable.

IMPORTANCE OF QUALITY SLEEP

When it comes to getting quality sleep during recovery, two things are true: (1) It's extremely important, and (2) It's going to be extremely difficult at the beginning. Sleep hygiene is essential for patients because good sleep is fundamental to overall health and recovery. Poor sleep can exacerbate stress, anxiety, and cravings, making it much harder for someone to stay on track with their recovery process. Healthy sleep habits help patients feel more rested, improve their mood, and enhance their ability to cope with the challenges of recovery.

Before treatment, many of my patients struggle with severe sleep disturbances. They often have trouble falling asleep, staying asleep, or have very poor-quality sleep. This can be due to a variety of factors, including the effects of substance use, withdrawal symptoms, and the psychological stress of dealing with addiction. As a result, they often feel exhausted and irritable and have a harder time managing their emotions and cravings during the day. As treatment continues, I see significant improvements in their sleep patterns. MAT can help stabilize their bodies and minimize the symptoms of withdrawal. This helps them to get restful sleep. Additionally, as they start to engage in healthier habits, like regular exercise and mindfulness practices, their overall sleep quality improves.

Some patients use meth to function when they're exhausted from a lack of sleep. They self-medicate their drowsiness and fatigue with the stimulant but end up creating a vicious cycle of poor sleep-wake behavior. When they first come off meth, it can be very hard to fall back into a regular sleep routine. They have to push through it with good sleep hygiene practices, such as setting a consistent bedtime, creating a relaxing pre-sleep routine, cutting out caffeine late in the day, keeping a sleep journal, and making their sleeping environment as comfortable as possible. These small changes can have a big impact, but sometimes, bigger changes are necessary. I once had a patient who heavily struggled with sleep because his work schedule was erratic. He worked days and nights on an inconsistent basis. Together, we discussed how finding a different job would help his sleep and, subsequently, his mental health and overall recovery.

Whether the changes are big or small, over time, patients who implement better sleep hygiene will fall asleep more easily, sleep through the night, and wake up feeling more refreshed. A lot of the patients just want to be prescribed sleep medication right after detox, but sleep hygiene and putting in the effort work much better in the long term. Like anything worth doing, it just takes time.

BUILDING YOUR LIFE BACK UP

Recovering from addiction often leaves a void in your life. When you get sober, you're going to have a lot more free time because you're not spending time either using the drug or engaging in risky behaviors that come along with supporting the habit. So it's essential to replace the void left by addiction with meaningful and fulfilling activities, such as work, social connections, and personal development pursuits. Building new skills and interests is vital in filling the new void. Discovering and developing hobbies, engaging in creativity, or pursuing educational opportunities can provide a sense of purpose and achievement, helping to replace negative habits with positive ones. I see the beauty of patients refilling their lives in positive ways every day at work.

Years ago, a patient showed up to his first appointment at Renew Health an hour and a half late. While we always try our best to accommodate these circumstances, that particular day was really busy, so we told him that he would have to reschedule for another day. Instead of leaving, he proceeded to have a full-blown temper tantrum in the lobby, put a hole in a wall, and lay down in the parking lot just yelling at the top of his lungs, kicking and screaming.

That was him back then. Now, he is one of my favorite patients. He's spent years working on his recovery, religiously came to his appointments (on time), and discovered a new hobby to help build back his life. He became enamored with spirituality, meditation, and self-improvement. Every time he has an appointment, he has a new book on the subject and is so excited to tell me all about it. He's doing awesome. The following patient testimonial is the story from the patient's perspective.

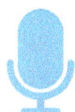

Rewrite Your Story
Testimonial from a Patient at Renew Health

I've struggled with addiction my whole life—even in my teens. At 16 years old, I started smoking weed and doing cocaine. Even though I came from a pretty good background, my dad wasn't around when I was a kid. Sometimes I feel like I didn't have anyone to show or teach me right and wrong, and that's why I went out to the streets, where I started hanging out with bad people and doing drugs. I ended up dropping out of school, and when I was around 20 years old, I got pulled over. In my car, I had guns and dope. They charged me with possession with the intent to distribute methamphetamine, and I went to prison for five years.

While I was in prison, I didn't really do anything. I didn't even get any tattoos. My mind was just so out of it. After I got out, I had my little girl. My relationship with her mom was rocky, and she didn't want a kid, so I ended up getting full custody of my daughter, and I've had full custody since she was a baby. I was doing well, in a new relationship, and staying off drugs. When you're doing good, it's so easy to say to yourself, "If I use again, it's just going to be one time. I can handle it." In 2019, I did cocaine. Once you pick up drugs again, you think you can control it. But when the next weekend comes around, it's so much easier to do more. Soon, it's every weekend, then every other day, and eventually, it's every day.

I was doing cocaine during that time because I didn't want to use methamphetamine. Cocaine could give me a high and a rush without the withdrawal, so I felt like I could be back to normal faster. But after doing cocaine for long enough, I started to need something stronger. Especially at work, I just needed something to keep me going. That's when I started doing meth. When the pandemic hit in 2020, I got laid off from my job, and my drug abuse got really bad. It was just like in my teens: Anything I could get my hands on, I was doing. Then fentanyl hit the streets, and bad turned to worse. At this time, my little girl was living with my mom.

I started running the streets again with my old friend who I got busted with when I went to prison in my 20s. We did everything to support our drug abuse: extorting, kicking in doors—just crazy shit. I started out just smoking fentanyl. I didn't want to shoot it up because I heard everyone was dying from it, especially when they were shooting it up. Eventually, though, I needed a stronger hit, so I was shooting it up too.

In February 2023, the guy I was running the streets with wasn't in my life anymore, and my girlfriend and I had split up. My mom would come over to my house, and she would say to me, "What the hell are you doing with your life?" I wasn't seeing my little girl anymore because I didn't want her to see me like that. To my daughter, I'm her hero. I needed help so badly. Every time I did fentanyl or anything, I just felt nasty. I went to so many places that turned me away. Renew Health was my last hope.

When I went to Renew Health for the first time, I didn't make it to my appointment on time, so they said they couldn't see me that day. I felt like nobody wanted to help me, so I completely lashed out. While walking out, I slammed the door and broke their wall. Then I just sat in the parking lot, crying and thinking, "What am I supposed to do? I can't do this by myself." After I left, Trent called me. With that phone call, Trent changed my life. I finally felt like someone cared—like I didn't have to recover completely alone.

It's been a year and a half since I started treatment at Renew Health, and my life has totally changed. The treatments have worked, I got a new job on a construction crew, and best of all, I got my little girl back. She lives at my house now, and she's my best friend. Now, I'm reading books every day on spirituality, meditation, and just overall healthy living. My mind feels like a healthy sponge, just soaking up everything. For me, I'll never go back to that life. They say "never say never," but I'm *done*. I have no urges, and it's not even on my mind. When I first started treatment, it was still on my mind a bit, but it's never on my mind now. It's crazy to me.

I look back at where I was years ago, and I just can't believe how bad it got. Sometimes I see people from that old life, and I tell them, "You gotta change, bro. You gotta get out of it." I always tell them about Renew Health. In fact, I would love to start a podcast to talk about this stuff and help other people. I know how hard it is to be out there, throwing your life away, hurting other people, and building up so much horrible karma. You can turn it around, but you have to want to. You can't hang out with the same people or do the same things. You have to be done with all of the bad influence and negativity. When I was using, I picked up plenty of bad karma. Now, I'm rewriting my story. I have so many plans for the future, but more than that, I have people who I don't want to let down. You can rewrite your story too.

This patient's journey is a story I cling to when I think about just how radically someone can change from their first visit. And it doesn't matter if it's meditation or working out or fishing or even fantasy football. It's important to know that there's a life after addiction, and it can be filled with as many amazing and fascinating things as you want it to be. The possibilities are endless because you won't be ruled by the substance anymore. You'll be able to choose what comes next.

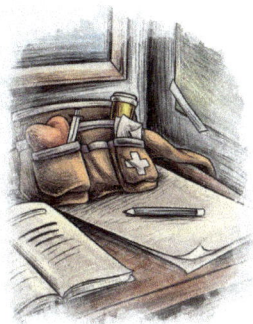

RECOVERY
WORKBENCH

Journal Prompts:

[?] What hobby have you always wanted to try?
- How can you take the first step to exploring it?

[?] When was the last time you made a new friend?
- Where could you meet someone new?

[?] What small things can you do to practice self-care?

[?] How can improving your physical health help you on your road to recovery?
- What are some steps you can take to improve this part of your life?

[?] What excites you most about the newfound free time you'll have in your recovery?

[?] What excites you most about the extra disposable income you'll have in your recovery?

[?] What are steps you can take to improve your financial stability?

[?] How would you rate your current sleep hygiene?
- What are things you can implement to improve upon it?

[?] Map out your current routines and the goal routines you would like to replace them with.

- What changes will you make to replace those former unhealthy routines?
- How will you stick to your new goal routines?

Current Routines	Goal Routines	How can you incorporate this in your life?

CHAPTER 7
TOOLS

☑ If you don't know what triggers you to take a substance, you'll never be able to avoid it. Once you are able to sit with your thoughts or talk to someone about potential triggers, you'll feel more in control when it comes to avoiding relapse.

☑ After identifying what triggers you, the next step is to strategize about how to manipulate your environment in a way that makes sense for your life. This could be as simple as taking a new route home from work or avoiding certain friends.

☑ When you have a medical provider who is on your side, they'll be able to customize a treatment plan for you that fits perfectly into your recovery journey.

☑ In the US, there are numerous different resources to turn to for 24/7 care so that you never have to feel alone on your recovery journey.

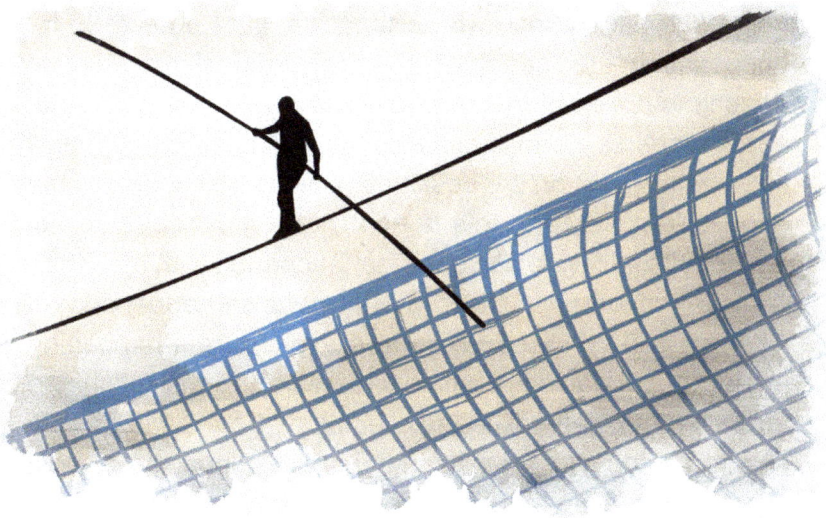

CHAPTER 7
RELAPSE PREVENTION

Patients often approach the topic of relapse with a lot of hesitation and fear. It's one of the worst-case scenarios when on the road to recovery. Even though the thought of it can be paralyzing, it's important to talk about it with your provider in order to prevent it from happening or to get you back on track if it does happen.

When one of my patients relapses, they are often hesitant to tell me. They might start by testing the waters with statements like "I've had a tough time lately" or "I slipped up a bit." It's usually clear that they're feeling ashamed and worried about how I'll react. I make it a point to create a non-judgmental space where they feel safe enough to be honest about their struggles. I let them know right away that relapse is a part of the recovery journey for many people, and it doesn't mean they've failed. In these situations, I help them reflect on the positives. They're still putting in the effort to recover, and this is especially shown by the fact that they're willing to discuss what happened with me. Then we talk about the logistics: why the relapse happened and what we can do in the future to prevent it from happening again. I understand that patients feel a deep sense of shame after having a setback in their recovery. Sometimes, a little shame can be a tool in preventing future relapses, but most often, I try to help them focus less on shame and more on self-compassion. How you move forward after a relapse is infinitely more important than the relapse itself.

The fact is, when patients come to their appointments after relapsing, I know they're already ready to talk about it. That's because at Renew Health, like most other clinics, the patients get drug tested before every appointment. Patients can refuse the test, but because I've worked to create an open and trusting environment, this almost never happens. After the drug test, though some patients still may try, there's really no denying the reality that they relapsed because I have the test results with me. Because of this, some patients face the music and immediately let me know they relapsed. I always try to let the patients be the ones to bring it up first in order to allow them to address it in a way that feels comfortable to them. But once it's out in the open, we are able to make a new plan going forward and adjust the treatment.

For someone who relapses on stimulants like methamphetamine, their sleep can be greatly affected by the relapse. Either they won't be able to sleep at all or they'll sleep way too much. It'll be a transition to get back on track and be able to, once again, sleep normally through the night. Luckily, the medication-assisted treatment for stimulants will not be affected by a relapse. The medication will have to fight harder against the stimulant, but the patient can continue to take the medication safely. On the other hand, if someone relapses by not taking their Suboxone and instead takes an opioid like fentanyl, the detox process must happen again before safely resuming Suboxone. Always consult with your licensed medical provider for guidance and supervision with MAT and MOUD. It's extremely important to understand the effects that relapsing will have on whatever medication you are taking. Also important is identifying the parts of your life that might trigger the desire to use again so that you can mitigate your chances as much as possible.

IDENTIFYING TRIGGERS

You can't avoid triggers if you don't know what they are. When in recovery, it is imperative to have conversations with your support group and reflect on what makes you want to use. I help patients identify triggers by encouraging them to think about their past experiences and current situations. It's a process of guiding them to recognize the patterns and situations that have led to substance use in the past. I often start by asking open-ended questions. Some of the questions I might ask include:

- Can you walk me through the last time you felt the urge to use? What was going on around you at that moment?
- Are there certain places, people, or activities that you associate with using?

- How do you usually feel right before you use? Are there specific emotions or thoughts that seem to trigger that urge?

These questions help patients dig deeper into their experiences and begin to pinpoint what triggers their cravings or urges. It's not uncommon for patients to initially disagree when I identify something as a trigger. For example, they might not immediately connect a specific emotion or social situation with their substance use. In those cases, motivational interviewing becomes a useful tool. I guide them to explore their thoughts and feelings more closely, helping them make the connection on their own terms. It's about leading them to self-discovery rather than imposing an idea on them.

The most common triggers I see are stress, social situations, and locations associated with past substance use. For instance, returning to a neighborhood where they used to use drugs or being around friends who are still using can be powerful triggers. Emotional triggers like loneliness, anger, or boredom are also very common. As for triggers people would not as easily anticipate, one that stands out is a patient who identified the smell of a certain type of cologne as a powerful trigger. At first, it didn't seem like something that would be associated with substance use, but as we dug deeper, it turned out that this particular cologne was worn by someone they used to use drugs with. The smell would immediately take them back to those times, triggering cravings and memories of using. It was surprising because we often think of triggers as being more obvious, like places or stressful situations, but even something as seemingly harmless as a scent can have a strong emotional connection. It's important to note that triggers don't always have to be only associated with emotionally distressing situations. Another patient realized that even positive events, like family celebrations or holidays, were triggers because they felt pressure to drink and use substances in those social settings.

If a patient has a trigger that they are unable to avoid, like annual holidays, that's when it's necessary to take the extra step and dive a little deeper. Checking in with patients about unavoidable triggers, like Thanksgiving, opening day of hunting season, and football season, means working with them to develop a plan when dealing with these occasions. I always think of the quote by Benjamin Franklin, "If you fail to plan, you are planning to fail." If you're going into a situation where you know something is going to make you want to use, you have to be prepared. This can mean always having an exit strategy, going places with a support system who will be there for you when these feelings arise, or even just making sure you're always holding a water bottle so that there is always something in your hand. It can be as simple as putting your hands in your pockets. For people struggling with alcoholism, seeing other people drink is a very common trigger. At the beginning of the recovery process, I'd say it's always going to be best to avoid any place where people are drinking. But once a person is more solidified in their recovery, going to a barbecue doesn't have to be the end of the world. It's important to have fun and live a full life. But it has to come with a plan, open communication, and mental preparation. If, after a couple of weeks, a patient still can't seem to be able to avoid the trigger, that's when cognitive behavioral therapy would again be a great place to work on day-to-day actions.

MANIPULATING YOUR ENVIRONMENT

Once a trigger is identified, learning how to cut it out of your life is a vital step in recovery. I call this "manipulating your environment." This involves making deliberate changes to your surroundings and social circles to support recovery. It can mean changing friends, switching jobs, picking up new hobbies, deleting phone numbers, or even altering the route you take to drive home. These changes help break old patterns and establish new, healthier routines.

When it comes to manipulating your environment, I believe it's important to balance both the immediate removal of triggers and the formation of new habits and hobbies. Initially, the focus might need to be on removing or avoiding triggers to stabilize your life and reduce the risk of relapse. However, starting a new, healthier lifestyle is equally important. Creating positive routines, like going to the gym, practicing mindfulness, or spending time in nature, can reinforce the recovery process and give you something to look forward to. In the long run, these new habits help you build a stronger foundation for your recovery. It's about more than just avoiding negative influences; it's about actively creating a life that supports their well-being and long-term sobriety. By tying in holistic healing practices with environmental changes, you can not only avoid triggers but also find new sources of strength and fulfillment.

I've seen patients make significant strides in their recovery by manipulating their environment time and time again. One story that comes to mind is a patient who realized that driving past the same bar every day on their way home from work was a major trigger. Initially, the focus was on simply avoiding that route to prevent the temptation. But as we worked together, we put a positive spin on it by incorporating healthier hobbies and habits. Instead of just avoiding the bar, we talked about how he could use that time to build a new, healthier routine. He started taking a different route that passed by a local park, where he decided to stop for a walk before heading home. This simple change not only removed the trigger but also introduced a positive new habit into his daily routine. Over time, this walk became something he looked forward to—a way to clear his mind and reduce stress, which in turn supported his recovery.

During treatment, I talk to patients about manipulating their environment very early on and readdress it if they come to me and tell me that they've relapsed. After someone admits they've relapsed, looking for new ways to manipulate their environment is a powerful way to keep the focus on the positive and figure out how to grow from the setback. I'll ask them questions like "Why did this happen?" and "What can we do differently?" Then, together, we build a plan to help them avoid that trigger in the future.

One of my patients, Melanie, has been with me for a couple of years now, recovering from a meth addiction. She's really putting the work in for her recovery, but unfortunately, she recently relapsed. She was avoiding her triggers and doing her best, but then her dealer knocked on her door and she felt caged in, so she used. When she told me about this, I said to her, "Okay, so this happened. You were doing really well. You were staying away from people, but they brought the drugs to you." Then I said, "Melanie, next time they come, don't open the door." Sometimes, manipulating your environment can be as simple as keeping the door closed on the right people. She contemplated the simplicity and said, "I never really thought about that." Even if some manipulations sound obvious, it's important to talk about them with people you trust because sometimes people looking at the situation from the outside will be able to see things more clearly than you can. It's important to note that when Melanie decides to not let them into her house next time, we're going to talk about that too. We talk through the wins just as much as we talk through the setbacks because there's a lesson in everything. You have to always look for ways to stay on course and mitigate urges to exit the recovery highway.

SUPPORT FOR STAYING IN TREATMENT

To give patients an extra source of help when in treatment, we have a patient success coordinator for them to turn to. Our patient success coordinator, Mara, is essential in keeping our patients engaged by building strong, ongoing relationships with them. She regularly checks in—whether it's through calls, texts, or in-person visits—to make sure patients feel supported and connected throughout their recovery journey. Mara also focuses on personalizing the treatment experience, tailoring plans to each of their unique needs. When patients feel like their care is truly customized, they're more likely to stay committed. Mara keeps an eye on progress, stepping in early if someone is struggling to offer extra support or tweak the treatment plan as needed. Another big part of her role is helping patients navigate any logistical challenges, like scheduling appointments or accessing resources, to make the whole process as smooth and stress-free as possible. By being that consistent, supportive presence, Mara helps ensure our patients stay on track and remain dedicated to their recovery.

To ensure the treatment facility you're interested in will be able to give you that extra support, it's important to ask. While we refer to this position as patient success coordinator at Renew Health, it may be referred to by other names like care coordinator or social worker at other clinics. When it comes to choosing the right clinic for you, ensuring they are able to provide you with medication-assisted treatment is essential, but asking follow-up questions about extra support, counseling, their ability to help with Medicaid, etc., is also a great way to make sure a clinic is best situated to help you in every single part of the recovery journey.

Mara works on patient retention. If someone misses an appointment, she calls them, checks in, and works to get them back on the schedule. On one occasion, when a patient was rescheduled because of Mara's check-in, that patient made it a point to thank her when she came in again. The patient said that if Mara hadn't called her, she wouldn't have come in. The patient even brought her dad in, who was struggling with schizophrenia and bipolar disorder as well as addiction. His name is Matt.

Because of Matt's co-occurring conditions, customization with his treatment was key. Mara is able to develop a relationship with the patients so that we can figure out the best way to customize their treatment plans together. Even though much of what was going on in Matt's head during our first visit was a symptom of his schizophrenia, it was reality to him. It was difficult to talk to him about treatment, so I asked if it was okay if I spoke to his daughter, which he agreed to. When I spoke to her, I told her about some referrals that I had given her father to help with his mental health and the two medications I was prescribing Matt that he needed to take. Also, I customized his treatment plan to include injections because that takes some of the accountability off of his plate since he wouldn't have to take numerous medications every day. For Matt, it was important to involve his daughter in his treatment plan, tailor his medications to his very specific needs, and work with our patient success coordinator to keep him on track with regular check-ins.

Customization like this is so important for addiction treatment. Everybody has their own little intricacies. Everybody has their own way of thinking, their own way of processing, their own triggers, their own environment that they're living in. So even though we have a standard treatment plan "playbook" for our patients, taking the time to make little tweaks here and there when it'll make a world of difference to a patient is a no-brainer. If a treatment center only works off of a generic script and refuses to consider the individual needs of its patients, the patient success rates will go down. When looking at treatment centers, ask the provider if there are ways to customize your own treatment plan to make recovery as smooth as possible for yourself. The only way to customize a plan is to let your provider or patient success coordinator get to know you. Open communication is key. Honesty is crucial.

When it comes to open communication, it should be available to patients whenever they are in need of it. At Renew Health, we offer a 24/7 call center, ensuring that when one of our patients wants to reach out, day or night, there will be someone on the other end of that line, ready to talk to them. This system allows us to provide continuous support and ensure that our patients feel heard and attended to, even outside regular office hours. Our goal is to offer reassurance and timely assistance whenever it's needed, making sure no one feels alone in their journey to recovery.

A 24/7 help center is crucial for a patient's recovery because it provides immediate support when they need it most. Recovery can be unpredictable, and cravings, anxiety, or moments of crisis don't always happen during business hours. The help center is used a couple times a week, especially during late-night hours when patients might feel most vulnerable. Whether it's someone needing reassurance, advice, or immediate support, knowing that they can reach out at any time can be a lifeline.

When a call comes in at night, I receive notice in the morning that someone used the help center. Then I make it a priority to follow up with them as soon as possible. I want to ensure they're feeling better and address any ongoing concerns or issues they might have. It's important to me that they know we're there for them every step of the way, not just during their scheduled appointments.

Many of my patients have really benefited from the help center. One that stands out is a patient who was on the verge of relapse late one night. They called the help center and were able to talk through their feelings with a staff member. That conversation was enough to get them through the night without using. The next day, we were able to adjust their treatment plan to better support them, and they've been doing well since. Another patient reached out because they were experiencing intense anxiety in the middle of the night. The help center staff provided immediate calming techniques and reassured them until the anxiety passed. The patient later told me that just knowing someone was there made all the difference and helped them avoid a potential relapse.

While some patients may turn to family members or friends if they're struggling late at night, sometimes people just want to talk to a professional or someone who doesn't know them personally. A help center is going to give an unbiased, correct response to someone who needs extra support. At times, even if a close friend tells you the correct response, it's not always something you want to hear from them. Calling a help center takes the emotional relationship out of the advice. If your clinic doesn't have a 24/7 help center, there are numerous free options available nationwide in the US.

- DrugAbuse.com hotline: 313-202-4254 – Addiction navigators are on call 24/7 to help answer any questions related to drug abuse and support.
- Al-Anon and Alateen hotline: 800-356-9996 – Counselors provide support to teens and adults who are negatively impacted by alcohol addiction and provide resources to group therapy nearby for ongoing support.
- Substance Abuse and Mental Health Services Administration (SAMHSA): 1-800-662-4357 – English/Spanish-speaking counselors provide referrals to treatment facilities, support groups, and community-based services.
- National Suicide Prevention: 988 – Support to help those in crisis process their emotional distress and prevent suicide.
- Boys Town: 1-800-448-3000 – Over 140 languages can be translated; they also provide a telecommunications device for the deaf (TDD) line for the speech and hearing impaired (1-800-448-1833).
- Drugfree.org: call 855-378-4373 or text 55753 – Counselors provide support and education and guide you to the best course of action.[1]

PATIENCE WITH PATIENTS

Every day at Renew Health, we strive to keep our patients in treatment, but it's important to note that every clinic is going to have its breaking point as far as what they will tolerate before having to turn a patient away. We try to be as flexible as we can be, moving around appointments to meet with patients as soon as possible while always following up when someone misses an appointment. But there has to be a balance. We've found that if we're too lenient with patients, some will take advantage of that and never show up to appointments or constantly reschedule. Also, patients might not take the process seriously, and they could start to slip into old habits or disengage from their recovery. On the other hand, if we were ever too hard on patients, it could create a sense of pressure, shame, or fear, which might push them away from treatment altogether. It would mean turning away a lot of people who are obviously in pain and seeking help. I've had patients tell me about other clinics that will automatically turn away people if they miss three appointments. To me, this is entirely counterproductive as it just reinforces the mentality that many patients have: "The whole world is against me." We try to find that balance by having our limits and being consistent, but always leading with understanding and compassion. Communication goes a long way. If a patient can't make their appointment, but they let us know in advance, then we do everything we can to reschedule. If they're running late but give us a call, we always try to work them back into the schedule. But if a patient no-shows without a warning and calls three days later for a prescription refill, then the answer is no. If they show up an hour late without first calling, they'll be seen another day. We have to support the patients who come ready to work on their recovery first.

In order to prevent turning patients away, we make sure to set these clear expectations from the beginning. Unfortunately, there is a very small number of patients who cross certain lines, leading us to decide that Renew Health isn't the right fit for them. This includes patients who rarely ever come to their appointments and patients who become violent, putting my staff in danger. We never want a Renew Health patient to feel abandoned, but we also need to strive to make sure treatment is available in a safe environment that suits everyone's needs. Sometimes, this might mean referring a patient to a more suitable program if we feel that's in their best interest, like a detox center or an inpatient facility. But ultimately, our focus is on helping each patient succeed in their recovery, and that requires finding the right balance in how we hold them accountable. Sometimes, if a patient isn't sticking to treatment when I'm only seeing them once a month, I'll switch to only giving them a week's worth of medication, requiring them to come back weekly in order to stay on track. Other times, the patient just isn't taking the medication as prescribed, so we have to come up with new solutions to help them. A great example of this is a patient named Emma.

To start her treatment, I prescribed Emma a month's worth of Suboxone. Instead of spacing it out throughout the month, she took all of the medication in the span of two weeks. She called the office to get a refill, but I told her, "You can come in, but you're not getting a refill." I didn't know how she was already out of her prescription. Emma came in for her appointment in tears, not wanting to upset me. She told me, "I feel like a failure." Then I told her, "Look, you're not in trouble. But the next week or two is going to be really uncomfortable because you're not going to have the medication. There's nothing I can do to help with that." Even if I wrote her another prescription, the pharmacy wouldn't have filled it because she took the previous medication in half the time she was supposed to.

Emma may have slipped up, but she didn't veer from the treatment plan out of malice or lack of caring. When I asked her why she took her medication that fast, she said, "I just felt so good, and I hadn't felt that way in a long time. I could actually clean my house. I could get up and down the stairs. I could get work done." She wasn't trying to get high off of the medication; it just made her feel better, so she wanted to take more to make sure that good feeling stayed. We talked about it and talked through it so that she is able to stick to the prescription timeline the next time the pharmacy fills it. We customized a plan to manipulate her environment and become more intentional about where to place the medication in her house. Since she is supposed to only take three strips of Suboxone a day, I told her to put three strips in her kitchen every morning and to leave the rest away in the bathroom. That way, she could keep track of how much she was taking every day and mitigate the desire to take more. Emma's story is an important testament to the fact that making a mistake in treatment doesn't have to be the end of the world, and it should never affect your ability to talk to your provider about it. Instead, it can be a time to reach out and ask for additional support. You'll find more compassion than you think.

Whichever step you're on in your recovery, whether it be recovering from a relapse, identifying triggers, or figuring out how to manipulate your environment, talking to your provider and your support system is a great way to begin to formulate a treatment plan that works perfectly for your lifestyle. Call a help center when you're feeling vulnerable. Reflect on how you felt before the last time you relapsed. Ask your provider if they have any ideas for how to manipulate your environment. There's no "one size fits all" when it comes to maintaining sobriety. Things that work for others might not work for you, but it's important to try every avenue you can in order to make your recovery as easy as possible.

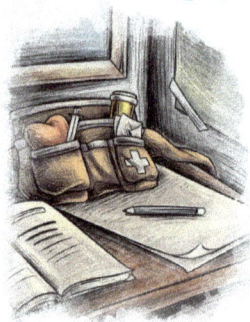

RECOVERY WORKBENCH

Journal Prompts:

[?] Have you ever relapsed or lapsed?
- What did you learn from it?
- What are you doing now to prevent it from happening again?

[?] What triggers have you been able to identify?
- Did any of them surprise you?
- How can you manipulate your environment in order to avoid these triggers?

[?] What does customizing your treatment plan look like for you?

[?] Have you ever called a 24/7 help center?
- How does it feel to know that support is there whenever you need it?

CHAPTER 8
TOOLS

☑ While on the road to recovery, there will be many different phases. It's important to learn about the different transitions and talk to your provider when you are ready to change your treatment plan.

☑ When you've been in recovery for a long time, it may become difficult to remember why recovery was so important to you. Staying motivated means remaining intentional and implementing new methods and goals when necessary.

☑ Whether you're interested in becoming a mentor or seeking mentorship for yourself, creating a community of recovered individuals can be life-changing and can make it easier to stay sober.

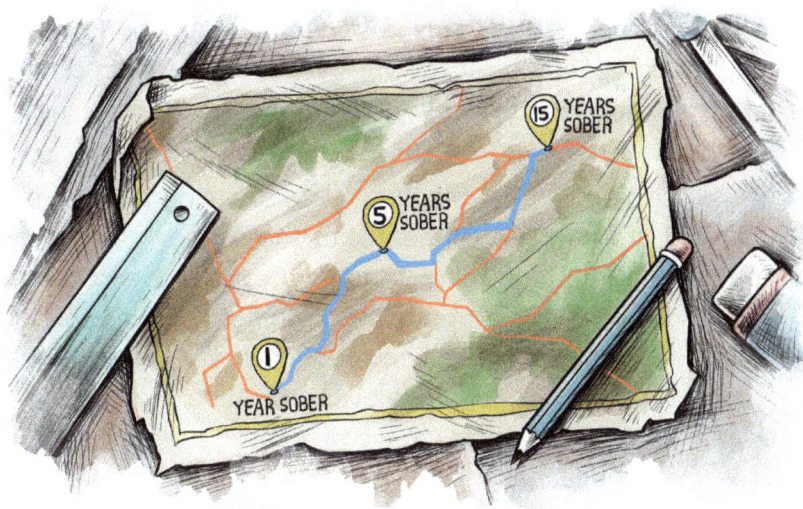

LONG-LASTING RECOVERY

When patients first start MAT, the road to recovery winds around obstacles, goes over bridges of support, and at times is washed out by unexpected storms. But as treatment continues, and patients are able to build their confidence behind the wheel, they stop looking in the rearview mirror and start to see a brighter future further down the road. They see their lives beyond the addiction they have confronted every day. Life doesn't magically get easier, but as patients commit to their recovery, all the skills and tools they've picked up along the way become second nature. Taking their prescribed medication, avoiding triggers, and remaining dedicated to goals may begin as road map landmarks that patients constantly refer to. But over time, patients don't need to look at the map as often. They know where they are going.

Maintaining long-term sobriety is a daunting task when a patient first starts treatment, but the further down the highway they get, the more capable they feel overcoming hazards that may have stopped them in their tracks before. What may have been a giant boulder in the road months ago becomes a rock they can drive over with ease. Roadblocks still present themselves at the worst times. It's unavoidable. However, the destinations further down the road are just too joyful and hopeful to give up on. Patients dig in and keep moving forward toward the life they have been working so hard to achieve. And even if someone gets lost along the way or does a full U-turn, there's always a way back to where they were going. There's always someone nearby to point them in the right direction.

My hope is that every patient is able to work with their provider to build a life beyond their recovery. With the help of medication, therapy, and a strong support system, I know it's possible.

A TRANSITION IN TREATMENT

Every patient's journey is different, but when the time comes, I'll start to meet with them less frequently. Appointments with patients begin with a weekly schedule, and as they become more comfortable with the medication and maintain their sobriety, checking in every week becomes less of a necessity. I make this clear to patients well in advance: Just because we aren't meeting every week doesn't mean I'm abandoning them. It's common for patients to feel nervous or scared during this period of transition. The idea of stepping back from a routine that began as the foundation of their treatment can be daunting. Those regular meetings provide a sense of structure and security. But when done properly, that transition becomes a milestone for patients. Moving from weekly to every two weeks to every month is growth—it means a patient is progressing and becoming more independent in their recovery.

I also emphasize that this doesn't mean patients are being "cut off." If they ever feel like they need more support, they can always reach out, and we can adjust the frequency of our meetings. If a patient needs two meetings a week, then we'll meet twice a week. One of my patients is on Vivitrol injections every month. She got to the point where we could meet every four weeks for that injection, but she requested to come in every two weeks. She wanted to be able to touch base in between injections and maintain that support. When she is ready, she'll take the next step forward.

Some patients are excited for their next steps and will communicate to me that they're ready to explore a greater sense of independence. They have to be truly ready though. A current patient, Greg, came in and said, "I'm ready to go monthly."

I had to be blunt. "No, you're not," I said.

Greg is a good guy, but as a patient, he's pushed the boundaries of our relationship. When we met more frequently, his drug tests came back negative. When we met less frequently, he started missing appointments. It's necessary we keep those weekly meetings to maintain accountability and build up a pattern of sobriety. The motivation to stay dedicated to a treatment plan should go beyond just promises. If treatment is disregarded or subverted, you run the risk of getting lost on the highway to recovery. But it's always possible to find your way back. And when you do, the rewards are only that much more fulfilling.

If I think a patient is ready to have less frequent appointments, it's because they have shown that they can be consistent within our clinic as well as out in the world. Those transitional appointments start with a negative drug test and end with easygoing, conversational check-ins. I watch as patients exhibit confidence handling situations on their own, using the tools and strategies we've talked about in prior meetings. When a patient discusses their challenges with more self-assurance, it's a strong signal to me that they're ready to take the next step. If that drug test comes back positive though, we have to reassess what may be going on.

Change can happen quickly, and even if a patient is doing really well, lapses do happen. A patient may be sober for six months and show all the right signs, but when they come in for their monthly visit, they test positive. My policy is to have the patient return in two weeks. Clearly we were doing good, but something happened, and now we're not quite where we want to be. If we get back on track, we can go back to monthly again. If not, we have to meet more frequently.

My patient, Chris, was having a positive response to treatment for about eight months but started using fentanyl again. Within a month, he was testing positive every time he came in. He moved slower, his skin was pale, and he had lost a ton of weight. He was scared and asked me what he needed to do. He was worried that his parole officer would drug test him, and he'd be sent back to prison.

"My advice," I said, "is to get ahead of it. Let your parole officer know what's happened, but tell them you're still coming in for treatment. We're working on it. We've got a game plan."

Chris was honest with his parole officer, and that bought him some time. But the next time he came into Renew Health, he tested positive for fentanyl again. As a last resort, I gave Chris tough love.

"Chris. If you don't get it together, you're going to be sent back to prison. Come on. Let's do this," I said.

Where we once focused on maintaining Chris's sobriety month to month, we went back to just getting through another week—and Chris did it. Since then, we've gone from meeting every week, to every two weeks, to every month again. What's most important is that Chris is still alive, especially with how dangerous fentanyl can be. It can be discouraging when you lapse and relapse, but that's never a reason to give up. It may be hard, but if you dig deep into what motivates you, you can continue to transition into a life beyond recovery.

MOTIVATION AND MILESTONES

It's easy to lose sight of how far you've come when you're in the middle of a journey. Keeping motivation up in long-term recovery can be tough, but it's so important to see success. I try to help patients stay motivated by reminding them of the progress they've made and celebrating the wins—even the small ones, like seeing me every two weeks instead of every week. As those wins accumulate, it's important to address any negative behaviors that have persisted. Addiction is a chronic disease that results in behaviors that become compulsive despite harmful consequences. When substance use is decreased, those behaviors can still remain. If your "normal" has been going through withdrawal, doing illegal activity to maintain your addiction, and finding new ways to get drugs, your reaction to a new, more positive "normal" is going to be eye-opening. Recovery isn't just about stopping substance use—it's about building a better, more fulfilling life. That new life has to be focused on your own personal goals.

Setting more audacious goals is important for patients to maintain their investment in their sobriety and keep motivated. Patients shouldn't be afraid to strive for bigger and bolder aspirations; just because a goal may seem impossible at first doesn't mean it can't be achieved. Goals help patients stay engaged and give them a clear marker to work toward. They are only effective tools if these goals matter to a patient, whether that's improving their relationships, pursuing a new hobby, or making strides in their career. When treatment begins, the goal may be as simple as staying alive—an important goal to have. Once patients start to feel the benefits of treatment, all the positive circumstances from being sober can snowball into greater changes. My patient, Ethan, is excited about starting his own company—there's nothing he wants more in his life right now. He's young, ambitious, and unfortunately, had a period where drugs were holding him back. He can now focus on his greater goals because of the freedom that MAT and counseling have given him. Goals adapt and broaden as a patient's mindset changes.

Patients who have been sober for longer periods of time experience their mindsets and outlooks shifting dramatically from when they first started treatment. Over time, as they build up their recovery and distance themselves from their old habits, patients start to think differently about themselves and their lives. This is often most noticeable in how they view challenges and handle stress. They're more resilient and more confident in their ability to cope without turning to substances. Patients will tell me how close they got to using or drinking and explain how badly they wanted it—but they didn't. And after a little time passes, they'll explain how much stronger they feel. Close encounters with substances happen, but if a patient is able to walk away maintaining their sobriety, that is a tremendous win.

One of the things I hear quite often from long-term patients is, "I haven't thought about using in weeks or months." Often, this doesn't mean that the urge disappeared completely. Rather, the urge has ebbed away enough that the patient can think about the future—what they want to achieve, how they want to live. This change in mindset is a major milestone in a patient's recovery. It's moving from a place where substance use is a daily concern to a place where it's just a part of their past, not their present. And they can now see that their future is full of limitless possibilities. It's truly inspiring.

The most powerful thing about when a patient is able to say, "I haven't thought about using," is that it's a sign that they're really internalizing their recovery. They're not just staying sober—they're living a new, healthier life with a mindset that supports that change. They've been incrementally moving their life in a new direction, and those short distances have finally added up to miles and miles of their recovery journey. It's important to keep this momentum alive. Sometimes patients need a little help to do that.

Having a strong support network is a big piece of the puzzle. I encourage patients to stay connected with peer support groups, lean on friends and family, and make self-care a priority—things like exercise, eating well, and mindfulness. All of these contribute to keeping their motivation up and their overall well-being in check. With the right support and a focus on both the big and small victories, patients can stay motivated and even motivate others on their journey to recovery.

SUPPORT AND MENTORSHIP

When a patient looks back on their recovery journey, they realize how many people have supported them along the way. There are many people who offer help and guidance, from friends, family, care providers, as well as others on their own recovery journeys. Hearing about another person's recovery journey is invaluable. It's more than just sharing stories; it's about sharing hope and strength. When someone who's unsure or fearful about starting their recovery hears how others have navigated similar paths, it can be incredibly motivating. These stories can be a powerful catalyst— sometimes even life-saving—as they prove that recovery is possible while offering practical insights and emotional support. To have a strong, diverse support network, you need to develop healthy relationships. Recovery doesn't happen alone.

Patients who are successful in their recovery have built networks that specifically support their sobriety. These are all the parents, brothers, sisters, friends, coworkers, and peers who want to see your success in recovery. You want the friend who congratulates you on being clean for a month, not the one who knocks on your door and offers you meth. It's heartbreaking to end relationships, but if you want to improve yourself, regain custody of your kids, or avoid prison, you can't turn to people who don't want you to make progress in your recovery journey. Finding real encouragement and motivation in friends, family, or a support group will be the fuel to keep you moving on the recovery highway. And when you get far enough along, you can reach out and help point the way for others.

Not Just a Recovered Life, but a Better Life
Testimonial from a Patient at Renew Health

I've been an addict since I was 15. Growing up biracial, I always felt empty inside, and I felt like I never belonged anywhere. I got into drugs and alcohol, and I even committed violent street crimes due to wanting drugs. The drugs gave me a synthetic high, which then gave me fake confidence.

Ever since I became an addict, I've been in trouble. I've hurt people that I care about. I've hurt my family. I basically just ruined my life. Even though I was good at sports, I would always be high at practice and games without my coaches knowing. It felt like I was living a double life.

When I got to New Mexico, I was put in a drug court treatment program, and since I was relapsing time and time again and overdosing almost every week, my coordinator said that the only options I had left were: (1) Finally die, (2) Go to prison, or (3) Try another treatment. That's when they put me in contact with Trent and Renew Health, and I started the Vivitrol treatment. I can't believe how much it's changed my life for the better. Now, my mom and I are doing good, my brother and I are doing good, and

I have trust back in my family. I also have actual, real confidence in myself. I just got my Class A CDL, which has opened up job opportunities, and I'm staying away from friends and relationships that I know are bad for me. Vivitrol has given me an opportunity to not only recover my life, but to live a better one.

I was always addicted to something, somehow, and in some way. But now, I'm no longer at my lowest point, and I can actually feel comfortable going into places without fiending or feeling like I have to get high. In fact, I never have a desire to get high anymore, and it's gotten me to the point where I actually have fallen in love with myself again. I don't think I've ever done that, even before I became an addict. It's a new experience that I'm very grateful and joyful for. I really think God put this experience with Renew Health in my life. And it's not only made my life better but my family's lives better. My mom won't have to go to my funeral. My brother won't have to go to my funeral. I can be an uncle, a brother, a nephew, and a good son. I can even be a mentor now.

I was basically nothing when I was in my addiction, and now I'm something. I'm somebody, and I'm going to do great things. I have a dream to open up my own rehab facility and get my doctorate in psychology to become a substance abuse counselor. And I wouldn't have done that without Vivitrol or Trent. It's just a greater life now, and I can actually live it without the heaviness or the burdens of addiction.

When you take someone under your wing, it holds you accountable. It's hard not to see yourself in someone younger than you, struggling with their own substance use disorder. Helping others only helps you. You may be feeling pretty confident and more solid in your sobriety, but someone else might need to tap into your strength. They might think about using and call you—and you can be the voice that helps them fight the urge. Mentorship builds out a legacy of recovery. A connected network of people who can support one another in holistic recovery.

My patient, Evan, talked with his cousin in Texas who has been struggling with alcohol. Evan shared his experience with MAT and how it's changed his entire life.

He told his cousin, "Man, I know you can do it because look at me. I've done everything there is to try. I've overdosed so many times. I shouldn't be here. Look at me now. Now, I'm over a year into treatment, and I haven't touched anything. I got my life on track."

Mentors are the physical embodiment of, "I recovered, and it's possible for you too." That kind of encouragement from someone who's been there can make all the difference in staying committed to recovery. While providers and family members offer invaluable support, a mentor brings something different to the table—lived experience. This can make conversations with a mentor feel more like talking to a friend who truly gets it, without the pressure that might come with talking to family or the formality of a clinical setting. This dynamic can help patients feel more at ease, knowing they're speaking to someone who has faced similar challenges and fears. Not everyone is lucky enough to have a sprawling network or a mentor in their corner though.

At Renew Health, we offer a foundation of support that you can rely on, no matter what. Besides my work with patients, our patient success coordinator offers even more motivation for recovery. Success is measured differently for everyone, so it's important for patients to be open and honest in setting their recovery goals. Our patient success coordinator checks in throughout treatment, shares encouraging words, and keeps patients focused on their goals. By tracking progress and helping set new milestones, the coordinator helps patients recognize their growth and stay engaged with their recovery. If a patient needs help, our patient success coordinator can connect them with resources, adjust their plans, or just be there to listen. We understand that sometimes you need to let someone know that you're not doing well. We make ourselves available because we know recovery can be challenging. But it's worth it.

We're a team dedicated to all the patients who come to us for help. We want to see our patients achieve their long-term goals. It's important to find a clinic that gives you the correct treatment while also taking that extra step of being committed to these long-lasting goals. Ask questions about mentorship programs or support groups that your provider offers or recommends. Having support and care that you can rely on is what makes long-term recovery possible. Medication-assisted treatment and its accessibility have grown exponentially in the past few years, making recovery a greater possibility for those affected by addiction. Dedication to your treatment and long-term recovery can save your life, and when you're ready, you can reach out and save someone else who is struggling on the road to recovery.

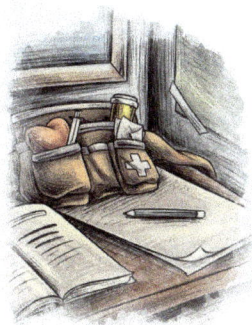

RECOVERY
WORKBENCH

Journal Prompts:

[?] What's your biggest goal or dream?

- How is addiction keeping you from achieving it?
- What smaller goals can you set to bring you closer to that dream?

[?] Have you undergone transitions in treatment?

- How did it feel to move on to the next step?

[?] Who has been your greatest mentor?

- What's a key lesson you learned from them?
- How can you offer help and mentorship to others?

[?] Write a letter to a younger version of yourself. Tell them about your recovery, what steps you've taken so far, and what more you have to do. Be kind to that younger self and be proud of where you are today.

TOOLS

- ☑ The fentanyl crisis in America needs to be addressed; millions of people are suffering every year.

- ☑ If the general public is more aware of addiction and recovery treatments, more effective programs can be put in place by local and national leadership.

- ☑ Addiction is a public health emergency and should not be stigmatized.

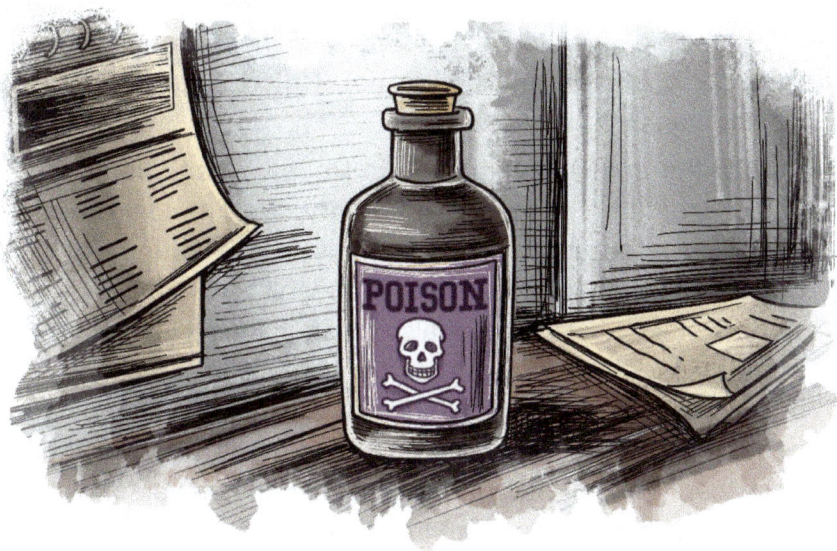

THE FENTANYL CRISIS IN AMERICA

A few years ago, there was a group of West Point cadets down in Florida, and during their spring break, they used cocaine. They didn't know it was laced with fentanyl. When four of them overdosed, bystanders who witnessed the overdose started doing CPR. The fentanyl ended up getting on their lips, and then the bystanders, who hadn't done any cocaine, went into respiratory arrest as well. They were just trying to save these young kids. Two of them were moved to the hospital in critical condition.1 These people were just trying to enjoy themselves on spring break, made a bad decision, and it almost cost them their lives and the lives of the people trying to save them. I wish these stories were isolated incidents, but they're not. Unfortunately, I hear similar stories on a weekly basis.

For the patients who come to Renew Health, fentanyl addiction is the most prevalent. Every day, I'm confronted with how large the fentanyl crisis is in this country and beyond. As with all addictions, it doesn't just affect those who use the substance, but also those in their lives: family, friends, loved ones, and even bystanders in the case of those cadets in Florida. Stories of these drugs harming people never leave my mind and drive me to continue the work that I do. For now, fentanyl is the most prevalent illicit substance in circulation, but there will come a time when a new substance takes its place, potentially even something more dangerous. Before that happens, we need to address the treatment available right now in this country.

Once we are able to put lasting programs in place, we can create an infrastructure that saves lives well into the future.

THE STATE OF ADDICTION RECOVERY IN AMERICA

Writing this book made me realize just how far we've come in terms of understanding addiction and recovery, but also how much work we still have to do. There are a lot of proven strategies and medications that can really make a difference, and it's frustrating to see that they're not as widely used or understood as they should be. With the effective medications we have available, I can change the life trajectory of someone who uses fentanyl. But for many, unless they have someone to walk them through what these medications are capable of, or have the word of mouth from a friend or loved one who has engaged with this type of treatment, their minds remain closed off to these options. The stigma around addiction and certain treatments, like medication-assisted treatment, still holds a lot of people back from getting the help they need. And with over 100,000 dying from overdoses in America every year, we have to act now to change the state of addiction recovery.[2]

Fentanyl is **50 to 100** times more potent than morphine.

Source: Center for Disease Control, Overdose Protection, 2024.

Source: Center for Disease Control, Stop Overdose, 2024.

Synthetic opioids like fentanyl contribute to nearly **70%** of overdose deaths.

42% of counterfeit pills tested for fentanyl contained a potentially lethal dose.

Source: United States Drug Enforcement Administration, Facts About Fentanyl.

Source: World Health Organization, Opioid Overdose, 2023.

Only **1/2** of countries provide access to effective treatment options for opioid dependence and less than **10%** of people worldwide in need of such treatment are receiving it.

At the same time, I feel hopeful. We've made some incredible progress in recognizing addiction as a medical condition rather than a moral failing, and there are more resources available now than ever before. But we need to keep pushing for more awareness and better access to care. Writing this book also reinforced for me the importance of getting the word out about what works and how we can support people in recovery—not just with medication, but with comprehensive care that includes counseling, support networks, and real, compassionate understanding. In the end, I feel a mix of frustration about the barriers that still exist and optimism for the future. If we can continue to educate, reduce stigma, and make effective treatments more accessible, I believe we can make a real impact on the state of addiction recovery in America.

Bringing awareness to the mainstream media is crucial because the media shapes public perception. And it goes without saying that while addiction is sometimes covered by news outlets, it's not always an accurate depiction of the issue. Numbers get fudged sometimes when people want to win arguments. Other times, only extremes are covered in the media, like the "fentanyl fold," in which drug users lose a degree of consciousness and muscle control.[3] While these images of people slumped over on the streets depict one aspect of America's fentanyl crisis, it's also important to report that people you see every day and would never suspect could be afflicted with addiction. Additionally, many public figures want to place blame on other countries like China and Mexico. Instead of placing blame and "washing our hands of it," we need to reflect on what we can control and improve within America. When addiction is portrayed accurately— when people see the stories of real individuals recovering with the help of proven strategies and treatments—it reduces the stigma that keeps so many from seeking help. The more the media shares about the effectiveness of medication-assisted treatment and other evidence-based approaches, the more we can shift the narrative from shame and judgment to one of hope and recovery. Awareness also drives policy changes and opens the door for better funding and access to care, instead of just locking people up who have a problem.

The public needs to understand how important it is to advocate for treatment over incarceration. Imprisonment doesn't address the root causes of their substance use—it just perpetuates the cycle of addiction with more barriers, especially considering how many incarcerated individuals struggle with addiction. In fact, according to the National Institutes of Health, "an estimated one-half of all prisoners (including some sentenced for other than drug offenses) meet the criteria for diagnosis of drug abuse or dependence." Of that group, only about 15–20 percent receive drug abuse treatment.[4] People struggling with addiction need medical care, therapy, and support to recover—not punishment. Incarceration as punishment just means there is no follow-through. Alternatively, treatment offers a path to recovery, healing, and reintegration into society. At Renew Health, I am always looking for ways to connect our services to those in the prison system who need them, whether that be telehealth visits, immediate appointments upon release, or anything else I am able to provide. By focusing on treatment, we give people a chance to get their lives back on track, contribute to their communities, and break free from the revolving door of the criminal justice system. This is especially important during the fentanyl crisis that we find ourselves in now.

The rise of the fentanyl crisis was shocking and terrifying to witness. The drug caused addictions and overdoses to skyrocket, quickly becoming the most dangerous drug in the history of the country. This fact is attributed to fentanyl's potency as well as the common practice of combining it with other substances, oftentimes completely unknown to the user. Communities and clinics were unprepared when the drug first became popular. Now, while there have been positive steps forward like Narcan, harm reduction efforts, and public health campaigns, the response doesn't feel urgent enough. There needs to be even more education, more access to resources, and the installation of policies that prevent this crisis from worsening. As the old saying goes, "An ounce of prevention is worth a pound of cure." The rise of fentanyl has shown us that our existing systems weren't ready for this level of danger, and while some progress has been made, we need to do much more to truly get ahead of it. If I could get one message across to everyone reading this book right now in regards to this crisis, it would be this: Don't take anything unless it comes from the pharmacy. In this day and age, there's no telling what's in the drugs people are buying on the street.

Making a real difference in America's struggle with addiction requires a multi-faceted approach that treats addiction as the public health emergency that it is. This crisis needs to be addressed at a national level. When we treat addiction as a public health issue, we focus on prevention, treatment, and recovery—rather than just the consequences. That's how real change happens. Access to treatment is a major piece of the puzzle. We need to make sure evidence-based treatments, like medication-assisted treatment and cognitive behavioral therapy, are available to everyone, no matter where they live or their financial situation. This also means treating the whole patient—integrating mental health services to address co-occurring disorders, like anxiety or depression, alongside addiction treatment. After the first stages of recovery have been initiated, it's imperative that patients continue to receive proper treatment and support.

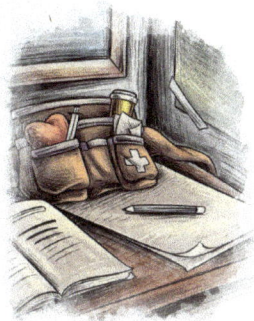

RECOVERY
WORKBENCH

Journal Prompts:

[?] Have you or someone you love been affected by the fentanyl crisis?
- What actions can we take to better address this crisis?

[?] What do you think are the biggest challenges Americans face in regard to addiction treatment?

[?] What do you hope for the future of addiction treatment in America?
- What steps can we take to make that hope a reality?

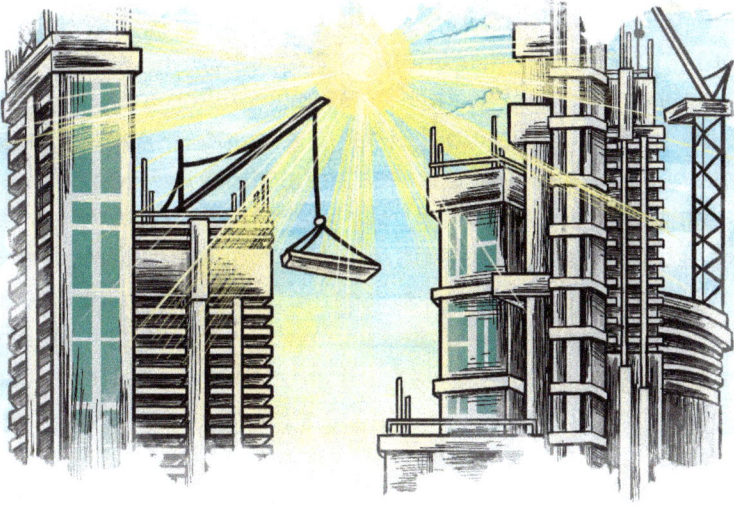

CONCLUSION

My dream is to have a solution for addiction for every individual in need. While this is a grand hope, I believe that many smaller steps can be taken to change the landscape and collectively lead toward this ambitious goal. These steps include increasing access to comprehensive treatment options, integrating innovative therapies and technologies, and fostering a more supportive and understanding society. By working toward universal access to personalized recovery plans and continuing to break down the stigma associated with addiction, we can make significant strides in transforming the future of addiction recovery. Collaboration among healthcare providers, policymakers, and communities is crucial to creating a world where everyone has the resources and support they need to overcome addiction and live fulfilling lives.

Creating a united front in addiction care starts with open communication and a shared commitment to addressing addiction as a public health issue. Healthcare providers need to be vocal about what's working—sharing data, patient outcomes, and success stories from evidence-based treatments like MAT. When policymakers understand the real impact these treatments have, it helps drive legislation and funding to support them. It's also true that policymakers need to consult healthcare professionals as well as community leaders when developing addiction-related policies because they are the ones dealing with the addiction crisis every day. This collaboration is key to real change.

In the same vein, community advocates are essential for bolstering local resources like recovery housing and other initiatives that create supportive environments. Recovery housing can mean different things, but it essentially provides people who are struggling with a place to live during their recovery transition—a place where they can have extra support, accountability, and stability before fully standing on their own. Measures like this would decrease the likelihood of people overdosing or freezing to death on the street. When all these pieces come together, we can create a system that prioritizes recovery, making it easier for individuals to get the help they need and reducing the long-term impacts of addiction.

In order to fully support patients, this holistic approach requires funding, broader access to centers, and laws that are focused on healing rather than punishment. It also requires other programs to be put in place to help patients secure stable jobs and teach them how to manage finances, giving them more reasons to stay on the road to recovery. Reducing barriers to treatment—whether that's insurance limitations or geographic restrictions—is critical. Dealing with insurance difficulties is by far one of the biggest roadblocks at Renew Health. At the same time, we need to reduce barriers for providers who want to treat this population. Incentivizing medical providers to get involved in addiction treatment will expand the reach of care, making it more accessible to those who need it most. Medical providers are already incentivized to focus on heart disease and diabetes, so why not addiction treatment?[1] Imbuing this area of medicine with money and incentivization will only help collect additional research and enable more people to help during this public health emergency.

In the end, these changes have to happen from the top down. It won't happen overnight, but little by little, progress means that in five years, we could find ourselves in a much better situation as a nation when it comes to substance abuse and addiction.

Every day, I work with people who are struggling, feeling lost, and wondering if they'll ever be able to turn their lives around. Yet, I continue to watch those same people transform, find strength they didn't know they had, and rebuild their lives. I chose to write *The Recovery Tool Belt* because I've seen firsthand how powerful recovery can be, and that hope is worth sharing with as many people as possible. I also wanted to share this knowledge in a way that feels accessible—a way that speaks directly to people in all stages of recovery, whether they're just starting out or supporting a loved one. Ultimately, this book is focused on showing people that overcoming addiction is possible. If even one person reads this book and is given a newfound sense of hope for their journey, that would be a huge win.

I'd love for readers to take action after finishing the book—whether that means reaching out for help, making a plan, or just talking to someone about their struggles. Because addiction tends to be such an isolating experience, I hope this book can help create a dialogue, allowing people to open up. I know that every part of the recovery process, especially detox, sounds scary; I want to share with readers that there's an easier path to recovery than they ever thought possible. There are people out there, many of whom I've met, who didn't think recovery was possible for them because they had been to 12 inpatient detox centers and it's never worked in the long term. I hope this book shows those people that if they've never experienced the continued care of outpatient treatment, if they've never tried medication-assisted treatment, their journey is far from over. It's just getting started.

Additionally, I hope that people reading this book learn more about how to find a good treatment center. A treatment center needs to be knowledgeable, but it also needs to make its patients feel supported holistically, beyond just addressing the addiction. So, when you get up and walk out of that first meeting with your new provider, ask yourself, "Did I feel like that person had the answers? Did I feel supported?" The key is to feel confident as well as cared for after meeting with a provider. If the provider is an expert, but they have a horrible bedside manner, it could still save your life and help turn things around. But the process would be much better and quicker if you felt supported because they talked to you for more than 75 seconds, intently listened to you, and took the time to give you an encouraging pat on the back.

If you're a reader who doesn't know much about addiction or who hasn't personally been touched by it, my hope is that this book opens your eyes to the recovery process. I hope you walk away with more empathy and less judgment, and maybe even feel inspired to be part of the solution, whether it's by supporting a loved one, advocating for change, or just spreading awareness about the realities of addiction. I want you to gain a better understanding of what addiction really is—not just the challenges, but also the strength and resilience that come with recovery.

Strength and resilience are new tools that everyone walks away with after recovery. Once you push through and achieve something you never thought possible, you'll be surprised how much your mindset changes. You'll be able to do more and won't be as quick to put limits on yourself the next time you find yourself in a bad spot. Pushing through hardships makes you stronger and gives you another tool to lean on when the inevitable next challenge presents itself. I have one patient, Isabella, who was absolutely paralyzed with fear when she first came to me. She's a woman who has been doing meth for practically her whole life. When she came in, she told me, "I know I want to change because I'm just tired of living like this, but I'm scared because I don't know what to expect. This addiction is all I've ever known." Now that she's in recovery, she has a brightness to her because she managed to conquer her fear of the unknown and make it out on the other side. The strengthening of mental resilience is an incredible collateral effect of addiction recovery.

It takes courage and dedication to pick up your recovery tool belt and get to work each day. You have to invest the time and effort into collecting all the tools you need for the job at hand and even learn how to use them. But once you do, you can build a life free from addiction with unlimited potential. Not everyone has access to these tools just yet, and we need to do better to help those who need it.

HOPE FOR THE FUTURE

The ideal future of addiction recovery is one where treatment is accessible, personalized, and free from stigma. I want to be a part of creating a world where addiction is treated like any other medical condition, with a focus on long-term recovery and overall well-being. In this future, everyone who needs help has immediate access to evidence-based treatments like MAT, CBT, and integrated mental health services as well as aftercare services too.

Another key element is breaking down the barriers that prevent people from seeking help—whether those are financial, geographic, or related to stigma. In this ideal future, addiction treatment is available in every community, and there's no shame or hesitation in asking for help. Harm reduction strategies would be widely available, and we'd see fewer people falling through the cracks because they didn't have access to the care they needed.

I hope to look back one day and see how far we've come. Even now, we have access to more medications and technology than ever before, yet rates of addiction and addiction-related death just rise every year. The medication-assisted treatments we have now are working phenomenally, but scientific improvements on the horizon are beyond exciting. Experts are working on longer-term injections and even implants to help people stay on track for up to six months and beyond. We also desperately need an FDA-approved medication for stimulant abuse. With the new information we gain year after year, we need to change the playbook accordingly to ensure every move we make is a step in the right direction, especially when it comes to emerging science.

At Renew Health, we're striving to build that future by expanding access to high-quality, personalized care across New Mexico and beyond. This care includes treatment for substance use disorders as well as co-occurring disorders; it's care we hope to expand both with more locations and through nationwide telehealth services. Renew Health will continue to advocate for policies that prioritize treatment over punishment and reduce the barriers to care for both patients and providers in a stigma-free environment. We're committed to staying on the cutting edge of addiction treatment and doing everything we can to make sure that our patients have the resources they need for long-term success.

Not everyone reading this book lives in New Mexico and can seek treatment at Renew Health, but please know that the right treatment center for you in your state is out there. Educating yourself is a powerful tool for your recovery tool belt, and just by reading this book, you have the tools to build something beautiful and long-lasting. It will require great patience as you take accurate measurements and follow the blueprints of your heart and mind, drive in all the nails to frame your goals and dreams, and tighten all the bolts to secure your sobriety. It is hard work, and you might want to give up when things feel particularly impossible. But it is always possible to build yourself a long-term, durable recovery. So buckle that recovery tool belt on and start building.

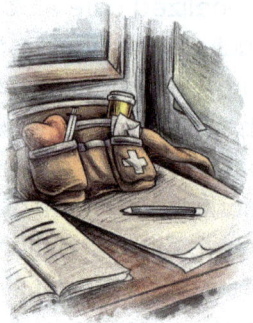

RECOVERY
WORKBENCH

Journal Prompts:

[?] What did you gain from reading this book?

- What did it change about your outlook on addiction?

[?] Is there someone in your life who would also benefit from the knowledge in *The Recovery Tool Belt*?

- How can you help others with what you've learned in this book?

[?] Why is addiction recovery possible for you?

ACKNOWLEDGMENTS

To my family—my wife, who has been my rock and source of unwavering love and support; my two children, who bring endless joy and inspire me to be better each day; my brother, who has been a steadfast friend; my mother, father, and step-father, who instilled in me the values that guide my life; my grandfather, whose wisdom and encouragement have been a constant source of inspiration; and my in-laws, whose acceptance and kindness have meant more to me than words can express. Your belief in me has been my foundation through every challenge and triumph.

To my close friends, thank you for your continued support and for being there to celebrate victories and navigate obstacles. Your friendship has been a source of strength and motivation.

To my patients, thank you for trusting me with your stories, fears, and hopes. You have taught me invaluable lessons and shaped my understanding of resilience and courage. Your journeys are woven into the fabric of this book and reinforce its purpose.

Collaboration has been essential to this project. A heartfelt thank you to Dr. Drew Fuller for writing the foreword with such insight and compassion, and to Dr. Bob Phillips for sharing your invaluable knowledge and perspectives. Your expertise has enriched this work.

To my dedicated team at Renew Health—your passion and commitment to supporting our patients fuel the mission and make a tangible difference. I am grateful for your hard work and shared vision.

To the support staff and publishing team, your meticulous care and attention to detail have brought this book to life. Your role has been indispensable, and I appreciate each of you.

To the broader community and readers, thank you for engaging and supporting those navigating addiction recovery. This book was created to empower, inform, and inspire a more compassionate world.

Finally, to everyone who believes in a brighter future for those impacted by addiction: We are all part of this journey. Writing this book has been a deeply personal and reflective experience, reaffirming my commitment to helping others rebuild their lives, find hope, and achieve recovery. May this book serve as a tool, a companion, and a source of strength for all who read it.

NOTES

Chapter One

1. Grace Sparks, Alex Montero, Ashley Kirzinger, Isabelle Valdes, and Liz Hamel, "KFF Tracking Poll July 2023: Substance Use Crisis and Accessing Treatment," KFF, August 15, 2023, https://www. kff.org/other/poll-finding/kff-tracking-poll-july-2023-substance-use-crisis-and-accessing-treatment/.

2. Kellie Schmitt, "A Brief History of Opioids in the U.S.," *Hopkins Bloomberg Public Health*, November 8, 2023, https://magazine.publichealth.jhu. edu/2023/brief-history-opioids-us#:~:text=It%20 took%20millennia%20for%20opium,babies%20 with%20opiate%2Dlaced%20syrups.

3. Johnathan H. Duff, Wen W. Shen, Liana W. Rosen, and Joanna R. Lampe, "The Opioid Crisis in the United States: A Brief History," CRS Reports, November 30, 2022, https://crsreports.congress. gov/product/pdf/IF/IF12260.

4. Joseph Detrano, "The Four-Sentence Letter Behind the Rise of Oxycontin," Rutgers–New Brunswick Center for Alcohol & Substance Use Studies, accessed November 21, 2024, https:// alcoholstudies.rutgers.edu/the-four-sentence-letter-behind-the-rise-of-oxycontin/.

5. Sari Horwitz, Scott Higham, Dalton Bennett, and Meryl Kornfield, "'SELL BABY SELL!': Unsealed Documents in Opioids Lawsuit Reveal Inner Workings of Industry's Marketing Machine," *The*

Washington Post, December 6, 2019. https://www.washingtonpost.com/graphics/2019/investigations/opioid-marketing/.

6. Carrie MacMillan, "Why Is Fentanyl Driving Overdose Deaths?," Yale Medicine, March 18, 2024, https://www.yalemedicine.org/news/fentanyl-driving-overdoses#:~:text=One%20reason%20is%20that%20because,the%20symptoms%20of%20opioid%20withdrawal.

7. Kellie Schmitt, "A Brief History of Opioids in the U.S.," Hopkins Bloomberg Public Health, November 8, 2023, https://magazine.publichealth.jhu.edu/2023/brief-history-opioids-us#:~:text=It%20took%20millennia%20for%20opium,babies%20with%20opiate%2Dlaced%20syrups.

8. "History of Meth," History.com, June 7, 2017, https://www.history.com/topics/crime/history-of-meth.

9. "Cocaine," History.com, May 31, 2017, https://www.history.com/topics/crime/history-of-cocaine.

10. "Powdered Cocaine Fast Facts," US Department of Justice, accessed December 5, 2024, https://www.justice.gov/archive/ndic/pubs3/3951/3951p.pdf.

11. Mark Keller and George E. Vaillant, "Alcohol and Society," Britannica, accessed November 21, 2024, https://www.britannica.com/topic/alcohol-consumption/Alcohol-and-society.

12. "Alcohol Use Disorder (AUD) in the United States: Age Groups and Demographic Characteristics," National Institute on Alcohol Abuse and Alcoholism, updated September 2024, https://

www.niaaa.nih.gov/alcohols-effects-health/
alcohol-topics/alcohol-facts-and-statistics/
alcohol-use-disorder-aud-united-states-age-groups-
and-demographic-characteristics.

13. Marissa B. Esser, Gregory Leung, Adam Sherk, et
al., "Estimated Deaths Attributable to Excessive
Alcohol Use Among U.S. Adults Aged 20 to 64
Years, 2015 to 2019," *JAMA Network*, November
1, 2022, https://jamanetwork.com/journals/
jamanetworkopen/fullarticle/2798004.

14. "Science of Addiction," Truth Pharm, accessed
November 21, 2024, https://truthpharm.org/
addiction-treatment/science-of-addiction/.

15. Andrzej Pietrzykowski and Steven Treistman, "The
Molecular Basis of Tolerance," *Alcohol Research &
Health* 31, no. 4 (2008): 298–309, https://pmc.ncbi.
nlm.nih.gov/articles/PMC3860466/#ref-list1.

16. "Definition of Addiction," American Society of
Addiction Medicine, September 15, 2019, https://
www.asam.org/quality-care/definition-of-addiction.

17. Stacy Mosel, "Is Drug Addiction Genetic?,"
American Addiction Centers, February 7, 2024,
https://americanaddictioncenters.org/rehab-guide/
addiction-genetic.

Chapter Three

1. "Everything You Need to Know About Substance
Use Detox," McLean Hospital, April 25, 2024,
https://www.mcleanhospital.org/essential/addiction-
detox.

2. "About Us," Alianza of New Mexico, accessed November 21, 2024, https://alianzaofnewmexico.org/about-us.

Chapter Four

1. *Clinical Guidelines for Withdrawal Management and Treatment of Drug Dependence in Closed Settings* (World Health Organization, 2009).

2. "Almost 90 Percent of People with Opioid Use Disorder Not Receiving Lifesaving Medication," NYU Langone Health, August 4, 2022, https://nyulangone.org/news/almost-90-percent-people-opioid-use-disorder-not-receiving-lifesaving-medication#:~:text=New%20findings%20led%20by%20researchers,evidence%2Dbased%2C%20lifesaving%20medications.

3. Marc Larochelle, Dana Bernson, Thomas Land, et al., "Methadone and Buprenorphine Reduce Risk of Death After Opioid Overdose," June 19, 2018, https://www.nih.gov/news-events/news-releases/methadone-buprenorphine-reduce-risk-death-after-opioid-overdose.

4. Ankur Sachdeva, Mona Choudhary, and Mina Chandra, "Alcohol Withdrawal Syndrome: Benzodiazepines and Beyond," *Journal of Clinical and Diagnostic Research* 9, no. 9 (2015): VE01–VE07, https://doi.org/10.7860/JCDR/2015/13407.6538.

5. Steven J. Weintraub, "Diazepam in the Treatment of Moderate to Severe Alcohol Withdrawal," *CNS Drugs* 31, no. 2 (2017): 1–7, https://doi.org/10.1007/s40263-016-0403-y.

6. Jonathan Avery, "Naltrexone and Alcohol Use," *American Journal of Psychiatry* 179, no. 12 (2022): 886–887, https://doi.org/10.1176/appi. ajp.20220821.

7. *Treatment Improvement Protocol* (Center for Substance Abuse Treatment, 2009).

8. Maranda Stokes, Preeti Patel, and Sara Abdijadid, *Disulfiram* (StatPearls Publishing, 2024).

9. Nick Zagorski, "Naltrexone-Bupropion Combination May Reduce Methamphetamine Use," *Psychiatric News* 56, no. 4 (2021), https://doi.org/10.1176/appi. pn.2021.3.17.

10. D. R. Wesson and W. Ling, "The Clinical Opiate Withdrawal Scale (COWS)," *Journal of Psychoactive Drugs* 35, no. 2 (2003): 253–9, https://nida.nih.gov/sites/default/files/ ClinicalOpiateWithdrawalScale.pdf.

11. Privia A. Randhawa, Rupinder Brar, and Seonaid Nolan, "Buprenorphine-Naloxone 'Microdosing': An Alternative Induction Approach for the Treatment of Opioid Use Disorder in the Wake of North America's Increasingly Potent Illicit Drug Market," *Canadian Medical Association Journal* 192, no. 3 (2020): E73, https://doi.org/10.1503/cmaj.74018.

12. "High-Dose Buprenorphine Initiation ("Macrodosing") for ED Providers," *Macrodosing Primer* (Meta Phi, n.d.), accessed November 22, 2024, https://www.metaphi.ca/wp-content/uploads/ MacrodosingPrimer.pdf.

13. "About Us," Substance Abuse and Mental Health Services Administration, updated November 1, 2024, https://www.samhsa.gov/about-us.

14. "About NAMI," National Alliance on Mental Illness, accessed November 22, 2024, https://www.nami.org/about-nami/.

Chapter Five

1. "What Is Cognitive Behavioral Therapy?," American Psychological Association, accessed November 22, 2024, https://www.apa.org/ptsd-guideline/patients-and-families/cognitive-behavioral.

2. Michael L. Dennis, Christy K. Scott, Rodney Funk, and Mark A. Foss, "The Duration and Correlates of Addiction and Treatment Careers," *Journal of Substance Abuse Treatment* 28, no. 2 (2005): S51–S62, https://www.jsatjournal.com/article/S0740-5472(04)00138-2/fulltext.

3. 2023 NSDUH Detailed Tables (table 8.42A; accessed February 6, 2025), https://www.samhsa.gov/data/report/2023-nsduh-detailed-tables.

4. Michael L. Dennis, Christy K. Scott, Rodney Funk, and Mark A. Foss, "The Duration and Correlates of Addiction and Treatment Careers," *Journal of Substance Abuse Treatment* 28, no. 2 (2005): S51–S62, https://www.jsatjournal.com/article/S0740-5472(04)00138-2/fulltext.

5. John F. Kelly, Keith Humphreys, Marica Ferry, "Alcoholics Anonymous and other 12-step programs for alcohol use disorder," *Cochrane Database of Systematic Reviews* no. 3 (2020), https://doi.org/10.1002/14651858.CD012880.pub2.

6. "Addiction Test," Mental Health America, https://screening.mhanational.org/screening-tools/addiction/.

7. "Naloxone DrugFacts," National Institute on Drug Abuse, January 11, 2022, https://nida.nih.gov/publications/drugfacts/naloxone.

Chapter Six

1. Keri Wiginton, "How Exercise Can Help with Addiction Recovery," WebMD, May 28, 2023, https://www.webmd.com/mental-health/addiction/exercise-help-addiction-recovery.

Chapter Seven

1. Cassandra Keuma, "Drug and Alcohol Addiction Hotlines," American Addiction Centers, June 5, 2024, https://americanaddictioncenters.org/alcohol-drug-hotline.

Chapter Nine

1. Vimal Patel, "West Point Cadets Overdose During Spring Break in Florida, Officials Say," *New York Times*, March 11, 2022, https://www.nytimes.com/2022/03/11/us/west-point-cadets-fentanyl-overdose.html.

2. "U.S. Overdose Deaths Decrease in 2023, First Time Since 2018," National Center for Health Statistics, CDC, May 14, 2024, https://www.cdc.gov/nchs/pressroom/nchs_press_releases/2024/20240515.htm.

3. James Ward, "It's an Odd Side Effect of Opioid Abuse: Why Are Fentanyl Users Bent Over. Here's Why," *Desert Sun*, July 19, 2024, https://www.desertsun.com/story/news/nation/california/2024/07/19/what-is-the-fentanyl-fold-how-to-treat-opioid-overdoses/74471357007/.

4. Redonna K. Chandler, Bennett W. Fletcher, Nora D. Volkow, "Treating Drug Abuse and Addiction in the Criminal Justice System: Improving Public Health and Safety," *Journal of the American Medical Association* 301, no. 2 (2009): https://doi.org/10.1001/jama.2008.976.

Chapter Ten

1. Carol Torgan, "Patient Outcomes Improved by Pay-for-Performance," National Institutes of Health, September 23, 2013, https://www.nih.gov/news-events/nih-research-matters/patient-outcomes-improved-pay-performance#:~:text=Pay%20incentives%20for%20clinician%20performance,amount%20regardless%20of%20patient%20outcomes.

ABOUT THE AUTHOR

Boyd, Texas, native Trent Carter has always been driven by a passion for health and helping others. As early as high school, he knew he wanted to funnel that passion into a career in nursing. After studying at Texas Tech University Health Sciences Center, Trent began his career as a critical care nurse, advancing into specialized roles before earning a master's in nursing from the University of Cincinnati's top-ranked program, where he graduated with honors. From there, he went on to become a full-time nurse practitioner.

Along with his master's, Trent also earned the following credentials: Advanced Practice Registered Nurse (APRN), Family Nurse Practitioner-Board Certified (FNP-BC), and Certified Addictions Registered Nurse-Advanced Practice (CARN-AP).

When he moved to New Mexico with his family, Trent immediately recognized a need in the community: quality addiction recovery services and resources for people suffering from substance abuse. Moved by the struggles of patients and the growing opioid crisis, Trent sought to create a recovery-centered approach that empowers individuals to reclaim their lives. Combining his experience as a medical provider, his expertise in patient care, and his entrepreneurial spirit, Trent made it his mission to combat the nation's deadly addiction epidemic in order to save his patients' lives, families, and futures.

His leadership and innovative mindset have earned him numerous accolades, including the prestigious Texas Tech University Health Sciences Center Presidential Distinguished

Alumni Award and Community Advocacy Distinguished Alumni Award in 2024, for which he was hand-picked by the university president for special recognition. An honoree of Albuquerque Business First's "40 Under 40" in 2023, Trent also earned recognition for his company, Renew Health, as one of the Best Places to Work in 2024 and 2025. In 2024, Renew Health was awarded the Best Drug and Alcohol Rehab Center in New Mexico by the Addiction Group. Additionally, Trent was named a "Top Family Nurse Practitioner" in New Mexico by Today's Nurse in both 2022 and 2023.

Since relocating to New Mexico with his family, Trent has made a tremendous impact on his community through his entrepreneurial spirit, launching initiatives that set the bar high for addiction recovery services. His vision continues to drive him to innovate, pushing the boundaries of what addiction recovery can achieve. His work is transforming not only his community but also the broader landscape of addiction treatment.

Follow Trent's entrepreneurial journey at
thetrentcarter.com

RenewHealth
Addiction Recovery Services

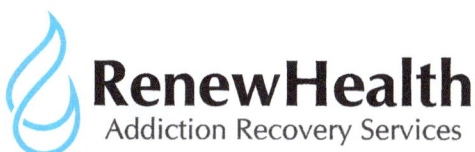

Helping people reclaim their lives from addiction

At Renew Health, our mission is to provide compassionate, effective, and accessible addiction treatment and recovery services. We understand that the journey of recovery is deeply personal, and we are committed to supporting each individual's path to wellness.

Millions of people suffer from alcohol addiction and substance abuse. There are countless lives and countless families ravaged by addiction.

Even worse, the problem is growing every year. We are here to do something about it. With our treatment methods, we hope to rebuild lives one family at a time.

For more information and resources, visit our website:
renewhealth.com